Autism Wellness Resources

Understanding the Causes and The Latest Non-Invasive Treatments

By Tony Meehleis, M.S.
School Psychologist

Table of Contents

Forward

As a high school psychologist, I was trained that once a child has been diagnosed with autism, specific learning disabilities, Attention Deficit Hyperactive Disorder (ADHD), and/or other various disabilities, they will have it for the rest of their lives...period. Approximately, eight years ago I started reading and exploring alternative healing modalities specifically for my own health issues.   I started seeing that private industries (Wellness Clinics, Natural Medicine Researchers) were finding therapies and solutions to autism and ADHD, but they were not getting any acclaim because these treatments were not "scientific and evidenced based." After much research, I felt compelled to write this book.

This research based knowledge has been a driving force for me, because I work in schools and see what is happening to children of this generation. Over the past 20 years, disabilities have gotten more severe, and more offshoot problems have developed in the average child.

According to school statistics, special education is growing at a medium pace, but the statistic you don't hear about is the dramatic increase of 504 (special accommodations) plans and students on home hospital. At a current high school assignment of mine, 504 plans have grown to be ¾ of the number of students qualified for special education.

I believe there is an epidemic of preventable childhood disease in America. One of the starting points of this epidemic is that government agencies lack control over what corporations are releasing into our air, water, and soil. The poisoning of our environment goes on from there and reaches into every part of our lives.

The target of this book is to reach people and parents who have used the medical and educational systems and have not seen the results they expected. They are looking for an alternative to the western medical model of using prescriptions, which simply mask the symptoms but do not heal the "dis-eases" or problems.

If you are among those with suffering children and are open to alternatives that are homeopathic in nature and non-invasive, this book may become your source for a wide range of treatment options, many of which most people have never heard or tried.

This research has been an exciting learning experience for me. I hope that you, as the parent of a child with a disability(s), will find some solutions to improve your child's life and your family's life as a whole.

Medical Disclaimer: This book is published in good faith and for general purposes only. A fair amount of the content of the research herein is not accepted by the American Medical Association and standard medical doctors. I recommend that you do your own research in order to make wise choices for your future. As I discovered, the answers are available.

Please consult a doctor before trying any recommendations, but be smart in choosing the right doctor – some medical professionals will not accept this research and these solutions.

Resource Credit Commentary: Most of the contents herein (aside from my own obvious thoughts and opinions) are taken and quoted directly from the sources acknowledged at the end of the book in the Resources section rather than within the chapters themselves in order to create easier reading. All of the contents are for public knowledge and are readily available.

Good luck. Tony Meehleis

Introduction

My name is Tony Meehleis, and I have been a regular and special education teacher and a School Psychologist for 20 years. I have written Individualized Educational Plans (IEPs) and completed psycho-educational assessments on a wide variety of disabilities that affect the children across our nation. During this time, I have seen firsthand the dramatic increases in children being diagnosed with autism, Attention Deficit Hyperactive Disorder (ADHD), specific learning disabilities (SLD), emotionally disturbed problems, and many other disabilities. When I was doing my MS program to become a School Psychologist, I was taught that when a child is diagnosed with autism, they will stay autistic for the rest of their lives, period; no cures or treatments are available.

Approximately seven years ago, I started reading books and articles about programs that were effectively treating children with ADHD and autism. As part of my inherent personality, when stimulated by a topic, I tend to open the flood gates to learn everything there is to know about the subject. I have spent hundreds of hours scouring the internet, buying and reading books, trying to uncover every bit of information on the causes of autism and their non-invasive treatments.

To my astonishment, I found that the private sector is taking the needed steps to create and use effective alternative treatments, and they are seeing results in children with autism and ADHD.

Peeling The Onion (uncovering truths)

It's been my life's mission to be on the cutting edge of new knowledge and research in a variety of subjects, especially education and learning disabilities.   When I realized that having autism may not be a life sentence, I started reading everything available.   It was like peeling an onion to get to the center.   The following statements will further explain the process of discovery and different perspectives on the reality of increased diagnoses of autism, learning disabilities, and other health problems in children.

Peel #1

First, I am familiar with "scientifically" proven methods such as Applied Behavioral Analysis (ABA), and they do have certain merit.   The direction I took for my research was "outside the box," and I looked for effective therapies that were successful but have not yet been recognized nationally.   Some creators of these programs were parents who had success with particular techniques on their own children.

Peel #2

Next, I pursued my investigation and kept seeing common elements between the articles and books I found. Toxicity and malnutrition seemed to be major contributors to many disabilities which are increasing in rate to, or near, epidemic proportions.   That led me to examine food quality and agriculture. I was shocked at the pronounced use of pesticides and herbicides and their possible connection to the increase of disabilities in the past 20 years.

Peel #3

As I continued down the path of research, I found the connection to Genetically Modified Organisms.   GMOs were quietly introduced into some of our major crops in the mid 1990's. The pursuit of Monsanto and other companies has infiltrated the entire food industry through genetically modifying seeds to be Roundup (a pesticide produced by Monsanto made from glyphosate) ready. The introduction of GMOs was supposed to increase output of crops per acre and provide a cheaper cost to consumers. The Federal Drug Administration (FDA) approved GMO use without any long term studies on the effects of consumption on the human body. Most European countries have banned the use of GMOs because of the strong indication of their harmfulness to health, but our government agencies refuse to pass even GMO labeling.

At the Core - The BIG Picture

For the last 150 years, America has been at the forefront of the industrial age; our advancements elevated a majority of people out of fairly primitive living arrangements. People evolved from living in survival mode by gathering, hunting, and growing their own food to farming with new cultural norms. With progress, people developed better quality housing, roads, and productive farms to feed the masses.

The overall lifestyles of the population of the U.S. rose dramatically. However, the upscale came at a cost that was not considered with the technological advancements that have rapidly occurred. The cost to the industrial society was air, water, and ground pollution.

This pollution was and is just a part of the toxicities to which we are all rapidly being exposed. The increased use of heavy metals, pesticides, herbicides, insecticides, and preservatives in vegetables, fruits, and meat sources, is corrupting our immune systems which can no longer handle the levels of toxicity.

Humans as a whole are getting sicker and sicker.   Sensitivities, allergies, and various disabilities are rising rapidly.   The younger generation's vulnerability to these toxins is way above allowable limits, and autism continues to rise and wreak havoc on families and schools. Even the older generations are suffering from this exposure with increasing numbers of people with Alzheimers, dementia, and other illnesses.

Are we now the "Toxic Generation"?

My goal is to write an easy to read but also comprehensive book so that others can learn about the crisis at hand and know practical steps to take to help yourself, your children, and grandchildren.

I am not a medical doctor, and my opinions and deductions are based solely on extensive research and discovery, all of which is listed in the

Resources section at the end. I believe people need to start a food revolution and learn what we can eat and what we shouldn't. We need to become aware of toxins, take steps to avoid them, and be wellness oriented so we can detoxify our bodies.

We need to take the reins of our lifestyles to change our lives for the better. We cannot rely on our government agencies such as the Federal Drug Administration (FDA), American Medical Association (AMA), etc., to protect us from pesticides, chemicals, and other products that are making us sick.

We must do it ourselves with our wallets and pocketbooks. We can stop buying products that are not healthy. Companies will stop producing and selling these products when there is no market for them. I hope you enjoy my efforts.

Premise

We are supposed to be Healthy and Well-Balanced in Body, Mind, and Spirit

Whether you believe in the Darwinian Theory of evolution (that we have evolved over millions of years from the smallest of cells) or if you believe in the Creation Theory (that man was put on earth as a whole being by God), the reality is that the human body is an amazing complex organ structure. We are near perfect in our function and genetic form (the majority of the time).

Yes, humans have abnormalities and genetic mutations, but statistics show they are present in only about 5 to 10% of humankind. Human bodies are designed to be healthy and last for much longer than statistics currently predict, even with new advances in medicine. There is an increasing awareness of preventive care and natural or holistic choices as well. However, lifestyle choices and environmental exposures to toxins and chemicals are altering the body's quality of life and longevity, and the results are increases in diseases, sensitivities, allergies, and disabilities.

Natural toxins have been around since the beginning of life; however, for the last 200 years, man has been tinkering with chemicals and chemical combinations with the hope of making our lives better. The materials we consume and are exposed to have been developed without regard for their long term effects on our bodies. In other words, without long term studies, scientists and the population do not know (or won't acknowledge) how damaging some of these products are and have been.

When people started to die from exposure to certain products, there came a new realization that marketing new products requires extensive study and research, which is unfortunately very expensive. We now know that some chemicals do not break down and lose their damaging effects for many years, if ever, and these toxins are commonly found everywhere.

Like most people, I was not aware of the effects that chemicals and toxins were having on the human body until I started researching the causes of autism. As I read hundreds of books and research studies, I started to see how massive this problem is, and that autism is only the tip of the iceberg.

Toxins poison the immune system which creates weaknesses that lead to inflammation in the body and brain. These symptoms bring about major ongoing health problems which then turn into diseases and disabilities. We are poisoning ourselves in many different ways. We as individuals, our government, and other supposedly helpful associations and corporations, are creating physical and mental problems which are hampering our lives and our children's generation.

The United States government agencies, with all of their policies and promises to safeguard us against harmful substances and carcinogens in the marketplace, are not protecting our environment, the population of America, and the world. If they can't or won't protect us, then we have to take action to protect ourselves.

We must take an "optimal health" point of view and limit our exposure to certain chemicals and products, taking the steps to rid our bodies and brains of these poisons. By becoming aware of the toxic materials and products on the market, we can stop purchasing them, which could eventually stop their use and production. These harmful products (noted in later chapters) are on the shelves of almost every store for all of us to unwittingly buy. I believe that we are at the very beginning of a Clean Earth Revolution, an Organic Food Revolution, a Natural Health Movement, and an Alternative Health Movement.

This book is designed to be a simple and brief guide to major toxins that are now affecting so much of the earth's population directly and indirectly. It reveals the connection between toxins and their effects on children. The focus is on autism and the epidemic increases in this disability, because it expands out to other disabilities and diseases in the young and old.

I hope to begin a rallying cry for a new revolution of people, government representatives and agencies, who expect and demand a healthy, nontoxic environment, and food supply.

Chapter 1

A Brief History of Toxins

The Chemical and Pharmaceutical Industries

The word toxin comes from ancient Greek and is defined as a poisonous substance produced within living cells or organisms. Further, toxins can be small molecules, peptides, or proteins that are capable of causing disease on contact with or absorption by body tissues interacting with biological macromolecules such as enzymes or cellular rectors. Toxins vary greatly in severity, ranging from minor (such as a bee sting) to almost immediately deadly (such as botulinum toxin).

The term toxin does not specify method of delivery, which can be from topical exposure to skin, inhalation through the air, consumption in food, or by injection into the blood system (such as venom). Toxins are simply biologically (in the original definition) produced poisons which can have little effect all the way to having major effects on a particular person or child. Herein, we will discuss and define only neurotoxins, because they have the most effect on the rise of autism, ADHD, learning problems, learning disabilities, medical problems, and troublesome behaviors as a result of exposure to them.

Neurotoxins are substances that are poisonous or destructive to nerve tissue. They are an extensive class of exogenous chemical neurological insults that can adversely affect function in both developing and mature nervous tissue. Common examples of neurotoxins include lead, ethanol (alcohol), manganese, glutamate, nitric oxide, botulinum (Botox), tetanus, and tetrodotoxin.

Neurotoxins can inhibit neuron control over concentration across the cell membrane, or communication between neurons across a synapse. Neurotoxin exposure can include widespread central nervous system damage such as intellectual disability, memory impairments, epilepsy, and dementia.

Humans have always needed to understand the hazards of the plants and animals they encountered or consumed. Early experimentation with plants was driven by interest in curing various ailments of the body and spirit. The father of Chinese medicine lived approximately 2695 BC. The Egyptians in 1500 BC wrote about anatomy, physiology, toxicology, spells, and treatments. A variety of poisons were used in early hunting for prey, war, and as a tool for suicide. As man progressed, so did experimentation with poisons and toxic materials. Most of the uses of these substances were not for good; they were developed for death and destruction of others.

Alchemy changed with the start of the chemical industry in the 1800's. The chemical industry transformed from craft based to scientifically based to industrial based. It changed from the 1850's producing dyes, pigments from coal, for textiles to producing plastics/celluloid in 1869. Then synthetic fertilizers were introduced in 1909. As the industry progressed, rayon from wood fibers was discovered in 1914 and nylon in 1928. The 1920's and 30's brought the rise of petrochemicals, and synthetic rubber was developed in the 1940's.

Today, the chemical industry produces over 70,000 products; most are not direct consumer products but rather consumed by other industries. We will discuss the toxic effects of some of these chemical products and their effects on the human body later in this chapter.

The pharmaceutical industry traces its origin to two sources: firstly, apothecaries that moved into wholesale production of drugs such as morphine, quinine, and strychnine in the middle of the 19th century and secondly, the dye and chemical companies that established research labs and discovered medical applications for their products starting in the 1880's.

In 1897, Bayer first synthesized aspirin which is now a household staple. Following over a decade of research, the concept that *synthetic* chemicals could selectively kill or immobilize parasites, bacterial, and other invasive disease-causing microbes would eventually support a massive industrial drive for research into new and easy-to-produce synthetic medicines. Shortly thereafter, the development of several important vaccines, including those for tetanus and diphtheria entered the market. Today, the pharma industry is one of the largest industries on the planet.

Consequently, today the over six billion people on earth are being constantly bombarded with chemicals and toxins from every possible direction and avenue. The chemical and pharmaceutical industries have tremendous influence over our government and massive power with their lobbyists. Unfortunately, they are producing more and more products that continue to have toxic effects on our environment and our bodies, which in turn, creates a worldwide problem.

(1)

Environmental Toxins

Heavy Metals

"Heavy Metals" include arsenic, tungsten, nickel, beryllium, antimony, platinum, cadmium, cesium, aluminum, lead, barium, tin, copper, uranium, thorium, mercury, and thallium.

Heavy metal pollution comes from the following sources:

- Coal burning, Mining, and Electronics

- Farming, Fertilizers, Pesticides, and Insecticides

- Household Cleaners, Plastics, and Toys

- Cosmetics, Deodorants, and Powders

- Medications and Vaccines

- Paints, Jewelry, and Ceramics

- Water, Air, and Food

These pollutions and toxins affect every living being. The severity varies depending on the location where you live, industries in the vicinity, volume of the population, toxins used primarily by that group, and even wind currents and weather patterns and how they affect the environment in which you live. Research has shown that the most far and desolate places on earth have the evidence of modern day toxins and pollutions.

We are increasingly being exposed to and poisoned by harmful substances every single minute of every day. The newer generations are the guinea pigs of our chemical, pharmaceutical, and agricultural industries. On a large scale, there has been no research on the long term health effects to humans on the new and varied toxins to which we are exposed. I strongly believe that we are seeing just the beginning of the overall detrimental effects. What lies ahead for the human race?

The focus in this section will be the effects of mercury, which is the second most toxic metal on earth (uranium being the first) and the one that is affecting the most people.

The association of mercury to chronic diseases is well documented in scientific literature. The National Library of Medicine's database for toxicology (TOXLINE) has reports showing the connection between mercury and cardiovascular disease, the number one killer in the industrial world. It also reveals mercury's association to cancer, the number two killer. Both of these diseases cause 80% of all deaths in the industrialized world. The relationship of mercury to neurodegenerative diseases indicates mercury's wide reach of impact on all humans.

How are we getting exposed to mercury? The main source of mercury exposure is silver/mercury amalgams in our teeth. This direct exposure can wreak havoc on health.

Mercury shows up everywhere; it has been found in soil, fresh water, and oceans. The marine and plant life absorb the mercury which is then transferred to humans from consumption.

Since the 1930's mercury was a main ingredient in thimerosal, a preservative used in some childhood vaccines. Since 2001, it is no longer used in children's vaccines, but it is still being used in some flu vaccines. People can request a flu vaccine without it. After it is in the human body, it can be transferred to a fetus through the placenta and mother's breast milk.

Some children diagnosed with autism also suffer from acute mercury toxicity secondary exposure while in utero. Mercury poison in autistic children is related to imbalances in body systems, including but not limited to significant allergies, infections, hormonal imbalances, gastrointestinal dysbiosis, immune dysfunctions, and nutritional deficiencies.

Children who suffer from chronic, insidious mercury toxicity secondary exposure over a long period of time may grow up to be adults who eventually get a diagnosis of Alzheimer's disease.

Due to our great exposure to it, mercury is the single most toxic heavy metal to humans; however, it is possible to avoid it.

Plastics

Plastic is everywhere, now in products that have invaded many, if not all, aspects of our day to day living. Plastic holds the food that is delivered to the market, and we also use it to store that food in our refrigerators and pantries. Plastics dominate the average kitchen and are in nearly every room of our homes. They are in every car and travel with us everywhere; in bottled water, in luggage, and even in clothing.

The toy industry is producing plastic toys faster than we can blink, and items, once handmade and natural, have been replaced with plastic counterparts. There is no industry, business, or home that is left unscathed; there are only a few diehard naturalists who refuse to use or live with anything containing plastic.

The invention of plastic in the 1960's has made our lives easier and impacted our life styles in many ways. Plastic is convenient and cheap; it has been fabricated into so many different products that it is nearly impossible to fathom how far reaching the plastic industry has ballooned.

An estimated five million tons of this endocrine-disrupting chemical were produced globally in 2008, and half of that was produced in the United States. The global industry analysts expect this huge production to continue to increase every year as more uses for plastic are found.

Sadly, the invention of this handy product has come with a cost, actually at a big cost, that no government agency or the plastics industry wants to admit. With all the good uses and benefits of this material, it can be harmful to our bodies in a variety of different ways. In this report, I will discuss only the effects of bisphenol, better known as BPA, a common ingredient in plastic which leaches into whatever it contains.

BPA is a synthetic estrogen that can disrupt the hormone system. The effects of BPA are just starting to be uncovered and revealed to the public. Effects are particularly evident when exposures occur while babies are still in the womb or in early life. Even minuscule exposures increase risks for breast cancer, prostate cancer, infertility, early puberty, metabolic disorders, and type-2 diabetes. Some experts believe that BPA could theoretically act like a hormone in the body by disrupting normal hormone levels and development in fetuses, babies, and children.

After a review of the evidence, the National Toxicology Program at the FDA expressed concern about BPA's possible effects on the brain and behavior of infants and young children. Some animal studies have shown a possible link between BPA and increase of cancer.

Studies have found that higher levels of BPA seem to cause a higher incidence of heart disease as well. Some researchers have looked into a connection between exposure and many other conditions, such as obesity, diabetes, ADHD, etc. More studies state that the chemical BPA is found in approximately 90% of all Americans.

The alternatives and solutions are as follows:

- Use BPA-free products (if they are labelled).

- Cut back on canned goods.

- Do not microwave of heat food in any plastic containers.

- Do not put plastic containers through the dishwasher cycle.

- Avoid bottled water or drinks whenever possible.

- Avoid non-stick cooking surfaces.

- Get rid of plastic toys that might be put in infants mouths.

- Use alternatives such as glass, porcelain, or stainless steel.

- Look for labels that read "BPA Free."

Building and Household Products

Every part of the structure of your house is considered a building product and includes the wood, drywall, paint, plumbing, electrical supplies, as well as the appliances and shingles on the roof. Most of the materials are non-toxic, but many times we are unaware of the ingredients in fire retardants, preservatives, or glues which were used in the production of these materials.

Most people are not severely sensitive to the products used in the building of homes, but some do have specific sensitivities. The two most potential problem products are carpet and paint. Note: This section does not include fungi or mold problems.

Here is a list of common household products that are made from toxic chemicals or have toxins in them:

- Cleaning products - ammonia, bleach, isopropanol, hydrochloric acid, sodium bisulfate, phenol, and lye

- Plastic - food storage containers, prepared food containers, and utensils

- Non-stick pots and pans

- Fabric protection sprays

- Cosmetics, deodorants, perfumes, soaps, lotions, and sunscreens

- Other toxins can include Radon, natural gas, propane gas, sewer gas, direct current (DC) magnetic, and electromagnetic fields.

Harmful ingredients in cleaning products can cause burns on skin, eye disorders, difficulty breathing, and lead to other health conditions, such as cancer, nervous system problems, and kidney damage. Bleach and ammonia release fumes that can irritate your eyes, skin, and throat. When put down drains, they can damage the environment.

In Europe, more than 1,300 chemicals are banned from use in lotions, soaps, toothpaste, cosmetics, and other personal care products. In contrast, the United States has just 11 chemicals banned. The average US woman uses 12 personal products and/or cosmetics each day containing 168 different chemicals, according to the Environmental Working Group (EWG).

Pesticides

Pesticides are chemicals used to eliminate or control a variety of agricultural pests which can damage crops and livestock and reduce farm productivity. The most commonly applied pesticides are insecticides (to kill insects), herbicides (to kill weeds), rodenticides (to kill rodents), and fungicides (to control fungi, mold, and mildew).

Agriculture accounts for 80% of the pesticide use in the U.S. Environmental Protection Agency (EPA) reports from 2007 stated that one BILLION tons of pesticides are used in the U.S. every year. This number is only 22% of the estimated 5.2 billion pounds of pesticides used worldwide.

Pesticides are not a modern invention; elemental sulfur was used by ancient Sumerians to protect their crops from insects, and medieval farmers and scientists experimented with chemicals ranging from arsenic to lead on common crops. Nineteenth century research focused on more natural techniques involving compounds made with roots of tropical vegetables and chrysanthemums.

In 1939, dichlorodiphenyltrichloroethane (DDT} was discovered to be extremely effective and rapidly became the most widely used insecticide in the world. Then in 1959, serious concerns about the human safety and biological effects of DDT led 86 countries to ban its use. The consolidation of farms and subsequent rise in industrial growing practices in the 1950's kicked off an era of heavy pesticide use.

There are over 350,000 current and historic pesticide products registered in the United States, and the pesticide business is a 12.5 billion dollar industry in the U.S. alone.

You and I have been lied to and deceived; we have been told myths about the needs of pesticides. According to the Pesticide Action Network of North America, these are eight myths from the pesticide/agrochemical industry:

Myth #1: "Pesticides are necessary to feed the world." We already have the ability to feed the world populations, and small-scale agriculture does not rely on pesticides. It is big agriculture conglomerates that promote pesticide use. Hunger in an age of plenty is not a problem; if we were serious, feeding the world could be done without the use of huge amounts of pesticides.

Myth #2: "Pesticides aren't that dangerous." Pesticides are dangerous by design and are engineered to cause death. Pesticides that harm human health are well documented; children and the elderly are the most at risk.

- An entire class of pesticides (organophosphates) has been linked to higher rates of ADHD in children.

- The herbicide atrazine, found in 94% of our water supply, has been linked to birth defects, infertility, and cancer.

- Women exposed to the pesticide endosulfan during pregnancy are more likely to have autistic children.

- Girls exposed to DDT before puberty are five times more likely to develop breast cancer.

- The World Health Organization (WHO) recently designated the key ingredient in the widely used herbicide Round-up as a probable human carcinogen.

Myth #3: "The dose makes the poison." Pesticide products typically contain several potentially dangerous ingredients. In addition, we are all exposed to a cocktail of pesticides in our air, water, food, and on the surfaces we touch, and the combination of these chemicals can be more toxic than any one of them acting alone. Many pesticides are endocrine disruptors and even at extremely low doses can interfere with the delicate human hormone system and cause life changing irreversible damage.

Myth #4: "The government is protecting us." Pesticide regulation is a fundamentally flawed process, and most of the data is supplied by the pesticide manufacturers. More than one billion pounds of pesticides are applied every year on U.S. farms, forests, golf courses, and lawns.

Myth #5: "GMOs reduce reliance on pesticides." Genetically Modified Organisms (GMOs) are driving up pesticide use. It is no surprise that the biggest GMO seed sellers are the pesticide corporations themselves. In 2009, 93% of U.S. GMO soybeans and 80% of GMO corn was grown from Monsanto patented seeds.

Myth #6: "We're weaning ourselves off of pesticides." Since 2004, the pesticide industry has had vigorous growth and continues to grow. Weeds are becoming more tolerant, and the use of pesticides is going up.

Myth #7: "Pesticides are the answer to global climate change." Evidence has started showing that *sustainable farming* without pesticides provides important solutions to climate change, with resilient systems that create far fewer greenhouse gases. But, as of 2008, pesticide manufacturers have filed for 532 patents for "climate-related genes," touting the imminent arrival of a new generation of seed engineering to withstand heat and drought (more GMOs).

Myth #8: "We need DDT to end malaria, combat bedbugs, etc." Studies have shown the use of DDT does not stop bugs and mosquitoes. Plus, the detrimental effects on the use of DDT have been scientifically proven, which is why it has been banned for 40 years.

Big agriculture now has little concern for the quality of our food sources and our exposure to dangerous chemicals. The representatives we elect need to become more educated about this problem and less influenced by the agricultural giants and lobbyists.

We need to work together to put pressure on politicians to curb the use of pesticides and promote appropriate corporate farming.

(1)

Herbicides and GMOs

An herbicide is a chemical substance used to manipulate or control vegetation and plants, and there are hundreds of different herbicides on the market. Some herbicides are selective and kill only certain types of plants, while others are non-selective and kill almost any kind.

Some herbicides kill weeds quickly, while others can take up to a week or more. Some herbicides persist in plants and soil for long periods of time, while others remain for shorter periods. Some have active ingredients that are more likely to move through soil towards groundwater, while others don't.

The potential effects of herbicides are strongly influenced by their method of application. Herbicides can act by inhibiting cell division, photosynthesis (amino acid production), or by mimicking natural auxin hormones, which regulate plant growth and cause deformities in new growth.

Methods of application include spraying on to foliage, applying to soil, and applying directly to aquatic systems. Some of the reasons for using herbicides are forest management, agriculture/crop cultivation, roads and rights of way, and weed control. They can be used in almost any outdoor space that has foliage.

I will discuss only the herbicide glyphosate, or "Roundup," because it is the most widely used and seems to have the most dramatic health effects on humans.

Roundup has been increasingly used over the past 20 to 30 years. It was developed by Monsanto, a controversial American agriculture company which has been at the forefront of producing GMOs and other poisonous herbicides. Monsanto has been claiming to help large and small farmers to grow food more sustainably.

However, Monsanto has a bad and long rap sheet and is directly related to the creation of genetically modified seeds that are Roundup ready. GMOs are the foods grown from these seeds. In other words,

Roundup is in the DNA of the plant, and its use is supposed to ward off weeds and insects to produce more crops per acre.

The FDA does have allowable limits to the use of Roundup, but many studies are showing that the harmful effects of its use far exceed the benefits. Independent studies on human cells and experimental animals have shown Roundup has serious toxic effects, such as:

- Roundup caused malformations in frog and chicken embryos.

- It caused birth defects in rats and rabbits.

- It caused total cell death in human cells within 24 hours at concentrations far below those used in agriculture.

- It is an endocrine disruptor and toxic to human placental cells.

- It irreversibly damages DNA which suggests it increases the risk of cancer.

- It causes disruption of neurobehavioral development, such as ADHD.

We are being exposed to Roundup in the air (especially in farming communities) and residue in the food we eat (if it is GMO or Roundup treated). The findings suggest that some of these harmful effects take place when the use of Roundup is far below the accepted limits that were approved by the FDA and agricultural government agencies.

Many researchers confirm that there have NOT been enough studies to show other effects and possible serious health risks which we are facing due to the increased use of Roundup and GMOs. The United States has approved the use of these products, whereas many other countries have banned the use of GMO seeds and crops and the use of Roundup by Monsanto.

Worldwide, 9.4 million tons of Roundup were sprayed between 1974 and 2014, making it the most heavily used chemical of all time in agriculture.

Additional Information on

GMOs and Roundup

A GMO (Genetically Modified Organism) is the result of a scientific procedure that injects DNA of one species into the DNA of a completely different species. This does not happen in nature and has nothing to do with hybrids. Presently, these GMO foreign proteins are labeled or banned in 64 countries.

In the U.S., 80% of our processed foods have been made from GMO corn, soy, canola, and sugar beets. Most consumers do not know what the GMOs are and in what products they exist, because the U.S. does not have labeling requirements.

The biggest corporate giant promoting GMOs is Monsanto. This company has been working on the "Roundup ready" seeds that can grow but will not be killed if Roundup herbicide is applied to them to kill surrounding weeds. No long term studies have been done on their effects to the environment and our bodies and organs. But yet, the FDA has approved their use in a high percentage of the vegetables that make it to our dinner tables.

Nancy Swanson, a GMO examiner and lawyer in the state of Washington *(gmofreewashington.com)*, reveals that data show correlations between increases in neurological diseases and GMOs, and the increased use of glyphosate (a broad-spectrum systemic herbicide) is the main ingredient in Roundup. Glyphosate entered the market in 1976, and its use has exploded since the advent of Roundup-resistant, genetically engineered crops in 1995. Roundup is applied directly to the soil and has been found in our rivers, streams, air, and rain.

The properties of Roundup disrupt the endocrine system and can lead to neurological disorders such as learning disabilities, ADHD, autism, dementia, Alzheimer's, schizophrenia, and bipolar. Those most susceptible are children and the elderly. There was an increased use of Roundup and GMOs in the mid 1990's, which directly correlates to the sharp increases in the autism rate which was initially blamed on vaccines.

It has been documented that the use of these products and their residuals cannot be washed off or cooked off and can remain stable in foods for more than a year, even if they are frozen, dried, or processed.

There is also a correlation between the more processed foods eaten and the higher amounts of Roundup in the bodies of the poorer populations.

Agricultural products are segmented into two groups:

1) those that are high-risk of being GMO because they are currently in commercial production.

2) those that have a monitored risk because suspected or known incidents of contamination have occurred and/or the crops have GMO relatives in commercial production.

High-Risk Crops:

- Alfalfa (first planted in 2011), a perennial flowering plant used for grazing

- Canola (approx. 90% of U.S. crop in 2011), the seeds used for coconut oil

- Corn (approx. 88% of U.S. crop in 2011)

- Cotton (approx.. 90% of U.S. crop in 2011)

- Papaya (most of the Hawaiian crop)

- Soy (approx. 94% of U.S. crop in 2010), used in food, oil, animal feed, biodiesel, etc.

- Sugar beets (approx. 95% of U.S. crop in 2010)

- Zucchini and yellow summer squash (approx. 5000 acres)

Monitored Crops:

- Beta vulgaris (chard, table beets)

- Brassica rapa (rutabaga, Siberian kale, bok choy, turnip, and Chinese cabbage)

- Cucurbita (acorn squash, delicate squash)

- Flax

- Rice

- Wheat

- Potatoes

Other animals and vegetables that scientists are currently tinkering with are tomatoes, potatoes, salmon, and pigs.

(1)

Insecticides

Insecticides are substances used to kill insects and include ovicides and larvicides used against insect eggs and larvae. Insecticides are used in agriculture, medicine, industry, and by consumers in products they buy for home and personal use.

They are claimed by insecticide advocates to be a major factor behind the increase in the 20th century's agricultural productivity. Nearly all insecticides have the potential to significantly alter ecosystems; many are toxic to humans; some even concentrate along the food chain.

Insecticides can be classified in four major categories:

- Systemic insecticides, which have a residual or long term activity; and contact insecticides, which have no residual activity. Furthermore, within these categories, there are three more types of insecticide:

- Natural insecticides, such as nicotine, pyrethrum, and neem extracts, made by plants as defense against insects

- Inorganic insecticides, which are metal

- Organic insecticides, which are organic chemical compounds, usually working by contact

Insecticides are commonly used in agriculture, public health, and industrial applications, as well as household and commercial uses. The USDA reported that insecticides accounted for 12% of total pesticides applied to the surveyed crops, and corn and cotton account for the largest shares of insecticide use in the United States.

A Brief History of Fertilizers

In the mid 1800's, England, was the first country to have a fertilizer factory producing superphosphates, also called acid phosphates. These comprised a water soluble fertilizer made by treating phosphate rock with sulfuric acid.

Germany later developed the famous "Law of the Minimum," which states that a deficiency in any growth factor (nutrients as well as water, light, etc.) will impair plant development. Replacement of nitrogen spurred the need for fertilizers. For this reason nitrogen, deficient in some soils, remained the single most limiting growth factor for crop production and stable food supplies until well into the 20th century.

Following World War II, many Western countries made food security a top priority. They set in place policies to encourage farmers to use fertilizers and other modern farming technologies. Fertilizer use grew rapidly in parallel with the growing world population.

The three basic plant nutrients, nitrogen, phosphorus, and potassium, became and still are the most used fertilizer ingredients on the market.

Our Food

Plant Based

Food is one of our most basic needs to survive. To start, we were hunter-gatherers by hunting for meat and gathering fruits and nuts for food sources.

Ancient people started farming to have more control over their lives and to grow food to store for the winter months. Farming gradually improved, and with the inventions of various equipment and farm machinery, it continued to increase productivity and output per acre.

Food used to be naturally grown and produced. After World War II, there was an increase in use of pesticides, herbicides, insecticides, and fertilizers. Our farms and food sources started to make a slow transition to increase output per acre. Most farmers saw the use of these pesticides as a way to improve production and make more dollars per bushel.

U.S. government agencies, such as the EPA and FDA, supposedly have control over the use of these chemicals by implementing maximum amounts that can be used on various crops. But has enough research been done now to know the long term exposure to these chemicals and pesticides on people?

The EPA states that it is safe to eat fruits and vegetables with a certain amount of pesticides on them. Here we are 60 to 70 years after initial pesticide use, and our farming food sources are tainted with the exposure to these chemicals.

These foods might even meet the EPA and FDA restrictions, but are those restrictions enough to prevent the proliferation of health problems and the poisoning of our bodies?

With the increases in food sensitivities, allergies, and other problems that are affecting the young and old, our government needs to determine if the use of pesticides is too harmful for our population.

- The fruits and vegetables highest in pesticides are apples, bell peppers, blueberries, celery, cucumbers, grapes, lettuce, nectarines, potatoes, spinach, strawberries, green beans, and kale.

- The foods lowest in pesticides are asparagus, avocado, cabbage, cantaloupe, corn, eggplant, grapefruit, kiwi, mangoes, mushrooms, onions, pineapples, sweet peas, sweet potatoes, and watermelon.

Go organic whenever possible!!

(1)

Our Meat Supply

Our meat sources have also converted to the corporate "production for profit" model. The meat companies and livestock facilities want to get the animals as big as possible as fast as possible with no concern for the quality of the meats and the additives used to make the animals bigger for slaughter. Here are some of the chemicals and additives in your grocery store meats:

- Antibiotics

- Growth Hormones

- Arsenic

- Feces of Other Animals

- Drugs

- Diseased Organs

- Pus

- GMO Grains

In addition, the facilities where these animals are raised are horrific, unclean, and inhumane. America's main meat sources, beef and chicken, are on a mass production line; get them big and fat as fast as possible; then get them off to the slaughter house. Other meat sources, like farmed fish, are equally as bad.

(1)

Processed Food Additives

Our food sources have made a major change since the introduction of processed foods in the 1950's. The majority of the population is eating foods that come in a box, can, packaged, or frozen ready-made. We live in a fast paced world based on convenience over quality.

Additives are put in to improve the look, taste, and shelf life of the so-called food. These additives cause us to consume more chemicals and less natural vitamins and minerals. In fact, some of the foods we eat have no nutritional value whatsoever. Listed below are the common additives you will find in processed foods and reasons to avoid them:

- Aspartame is a neurotoxin and carcinogen.

- Fructose corn syrup contributes to obesity and diabetes.

- Monosodium glutamate (MSG) is an excite-toxin and causes obesity.

- Trans fat causes inflammation and diabetes.

- Food dyes are linked to ADHD and contribute to cancer.

- Sodium sulphate contributes to asthma, headaches and rashes.

- Sodium nitrates/nitrites are possible cancer causes.

- Butylated hydroxyanisole (BHA) and Butylated hydroxytoluene (BHT) have neurological effects.

- Sulphur dioxide causes asthma and bronchial problems.

- Potassium Bromate has possible cancer links.

NIP is an acronym for food scoring factors. Consider these 3 things before consuming foods: Nutritional concerns, Ingredient concerns, and Processing concerns.

A final blemish to mention in the processed food system is "food irradiation," a new process intended to kill harmful bacteria, but it damages the few vitamins, enzymes, and minerals left in this fake food.

(1)

Our Water

America is running out of fresh clean water. Of course, we need to recycle our water and run it through treatment plants. The levels of particulates that meet government regulations are passable by some standards, but why do treatment facilities add chlorine and fluoride? Medical agencies say the use of fluoride is to prevent tooth decay and cavities, but is it really that effective?

What is really happening? Sodium fluoride has been added to the majority of municipal water systems since the 1950's. Sodium fluoride is also registered with the EPA as a rat poison. There has been considerable research done on fluoride regarding cancer, birth defects, and risks to the respiratory, gastrointestinal, and urinary systems. However, very little research has been done on its neurological effects and risks to women during pregnancy. A recent study shows a link between dental fluorosis and IQ damage in children (a decrease of an average drop of 7 points).

There are now over 100 animal studies and over 43 human studies proving fluoride's neurotoxicity. One analysis links fluoridation to ADHD in the United States. This report was published in February, 2015, in the *Journal of Environmental Health*. The prevalence of artificial water fluoridation in 1992 significantly positively predicted the rise of ADHD and other diseases in children and adults.

If it is affecting us neurologically, then why is our government continuing to require its use in approximately 99% of drinking water across the nation? Americans are over-exposed to fluoride at a mere 0.7 ppm level. What are other long term effects of fluoride treatment? Only time will tell.

An article written by Dr. David Kennedy DDS, titled "Scientific Facts on the Biological Effects of Fluorides," states:

- Fluoride exposure disrupts the synthesis of collagen and leads to the breakdown of collagen in bone, tendon, muscle, skin, cartilage, lungs, kidney, and trachea.

- Fluoride stimulates granule formation and oxygen consumption in white blood cells.

- Fluoride depletes the energy reserves and the ability of the white blood cells to function properly.

- Fluoride inhibits antibody formation in the blood.

- Fluoride depresses thyroid activity.

- Fluoride has a disruptive effect on the various tissues in the body.

- Fluoride promotes development of bone cancer.

- Fluoride causes premature aging of the human body.

- Fluoride ingestion from mouth rinses and dentifrices in children is extremely hazardous to biological development, life span, and general health.

- Fluoride diminishes the intelligence capability of the human brain.

- Fluoride studies in rats can be indicative of a potential for motor disruption, intelligence deficits, and learning disabilities in humans.

- Fluoride accumulates in the brain over time to reach neurologically harmful levels.

- Fluorides are general photo plasma poisons, with the capacity to modify the metabolism of cells by inhibiting certain enzymes.

- Drinking water containing as little as 1.2 ppm fluoride will cause developmental disturbances.

Adding fluoride to our water supply without population consent is a presumptuous and forced impingement upon our health, and government should stop immediately. The rationalizations and documentations the government uses makes one wonder what is going on behind the scenes. At this point, our only recourse is to avoid tap water by purchasing pure water or buy filtering systems for our homes, which have their own sets of problems.

For more information, please visit: *flouridealert.org*.

The Air We Breath

A recent study has found that over two million deaths occur each year as a direct result of air pollution. The Organization for Economic Cooperation and Development (OECD) issued a report that estimated the number of premature deaths from exposure to particulate matter (PM) is likely to more than double to 3.6 million in 2050, mostly in China and India. There seems to be a direct correlation between childhood asthma and other debilitating conditions linked to air pollution.

The American Heart Association reports, "environmental air pollutants that include carbon monoxide, oxides of nitrogen, sulfur dioxide, ozone, lead, and particulate matter...are associated with increased hospitalization and mortality due to cardiovascular disease. Although air pollution is a major environmental health problem affecting everyone worldwide, the most vulnerable are the elderly, the poor, and children.

Childhood asthma is on the rise. Asthma is a reversible obstructive lung disease that causes wheezing, breathlessness, chest tightness, and coughing. Currently, 9.5 percent of all children have asthma, an almost 50 percent increase from 2001 to 2009."

By adding air pollutants to all the other toxins and poisons to which children are being exposed and combining these with other co-morbid conditions, the results ensure a very unhealthy child or adult.

Biotoxins

Biotoxins are substances that are both toxic and have a biological origin. They come in a variety of different forms and can be produced by nearly every type of living organism. There are mycotoxins (made from fungi), zootoxins (made from animals), and phototoxins (made from plants). They can also be administered in many ways, including orally ingested, injected as venom, or released into the environment via spores.

Many biotoxins can be further classified by the kinds of effects they have on the body. Some of these groups include:

- Necrotoxins: substances that cause tissue destruction via cell death and are carried in the bloodstream

- Neurotoxins: substances that affect the nervous system

- Hemotoxins: substances that are carried in the bloodstream and l target red blood cells

- Mycotoxins: substances produced by fungi

- Cyanotoxins: substances produced by bacteria (also known as blue-green algae

- Apitoxins: honey bee venom injected via bee sting

Any biotoxins that are a threat to human health are classified as biological hazards. Effects start when a person is exposed to the biotoxin. In most, people, the biotoxin is "tagged" and identified by the body's immune system and is broken down and removed from the blood by the liver.

However, some individuals do not have the immune response genes that are required to eventually form an antibody to a given foreign antigen. In these cases, it will remain in the body indefinitely, free to circulate and wreak havoc. Once present in the body, the biotoxins begin to set off a complex cascade of biochemical events. The biotoxins that people need to be most aware of are neurotoxins and mycotoxins: for example, bee stings and nuts.

(1)

Vaccines

Vaccines have been the most controversial possible cause of autism for the past 20 years. Defended by the pharmaceutical industries and government agencies such as the FDA, CDC and AMA, it's no wonder the public is confused. A generation ago in the 1950's, children were given 8 vaccines from birth to age 18. In 2016, the number of vaccines required has spiraled to over 60 per child from birth to age 18, not including flu vaccine shots.

The first and biggest connection of vaccines to autism was the use of thimerosal, a mercury based preservative. Substantial evidence showed a direct correlation between the use of thimerosal and the rise of autism in the mid-1990's. The effects on newborns were staggering, terrible, and well documented.

A possible secondary connection appeared to be the increase in the number of vaccines required by the government and schools. To meet the requirements, doctors are giving multiples of vaccines in one shot and giving shots multiple times.

There are many case studies showing a regression in a child's behavior starting shortly after a vaccine dosage, specifically the measles, mumps, and rubella (MMR) shot at the age of 2 years old. Parents have documented that their child's health issues usually began with a high fever shortly after a vaccine shot and progressively got worse. Parents noticed the regression in a variety of human functions, such as speech, expression, eye contact, etc.

Patrick Timpone's, One Radio Network, published an article in 2016 titled, *30 Scientific Studies That Prove Vaccines Cause Autism*, which used data from mainstream medical journals whose studies verify the validity of the connection between autism and vaccines.

I strongly believe that all parents need to question the recommended vaccine schedule by doing research and discussing the various options with their pediatricians. Parents need to be more proactive in decisions made for their children. Their freedom includes choice of which vaccines are to be given to their children with the option of spreading them out over a period of time.

Avoiding MEGA vaccinations is also something to consider with the doctor. The other option is to avoid vaccinations altogether for your children, which is getting harder and harder to do, because states have been passing mandatory vaccination laws which negate the opt-out clause.

(1)

Electromagnetic Fields (EMFs)

In the last 150 years, electricity has become an essential part of our lives and was one of the most important factors that fueled the Industrial Revolution. However, there is a health cost with the increase in exposure to it as we are bombarded with electrical frequencies in various forms every second of every day.

The five sources of electromagnetic field exposure are:

- Electric fields are emitted from anything that has voltage and includes lamps, wiring, extension cords, appliances, power lines, and outlets.

- Magnetic fields are the main components of most motors that are in appliances such as refrigerators, etc.

- Power lines are above or below ground.

- Metal plumbing also carries a current.

- Wireless technology because it is everywhere from cell towers, wireless modems, printers, and smart meters.

We are continually being exposed to frequencies which we can't see, touch, hear, taste, or smell - 24 hours a day. Numerous health problems are being connected to this electro-exposure such as certain types of cancers along with subtle effects such as fatigue, headaches, depression, and sleep problems. We need to minimize our exposure, but how? Here are some things to consider:

- Cell phones: Use only the speaker or earbuds; do not put up to your head.

- Consider turning off wireless monitors at night.

- Turn off and unplug all motors when possible.

- Replace your smart meter on the electric line (if you can).

Chapter 2

Autism - Our Children Are Becoming Toxic and Poisoned

As explained in Chapter 1, our bodies are being hit from every direction with toxins. The slow and mounting process of toxic exposure affects everyone in varying degrees.   Since conception, the toxins in a mother are transferred to the fetus through   blood connection via the placenta. Within the first few hours after birth, doctors begin the never ending barrage of vaccines that have all sorts of chemical and heavy metal preservatives.   Currently, the total number of vaccines given to the majority of the population is close to 70 by the time a child is 18 years old!

We continue to breathe in air pollution and drink poorly processed water with fluorides and other contaminants. Babies eat processed baby food with high concentrations of sugar and other additives and drink soy derived formula milk.

As children get older, they eat pesticide and herbicide tainted vegetables and processed meat that has ingested antibiotics, steroids, and growth stimulating hormones. As a child starts to crawl and move about the home, there is exposure to household products found everywhere from the carpet flooring to the paint on the walls, to soaps, sprays, and detergents.

Kids eat and drink out of plastic containers that are made with BPA (a controversial chemical), and parents cook with cookware that sheds Teflon surfaces into the meals. As they age, children are bombarded with wireless and cell phone frequencies and use phones that emit radiation.

The furniture they sit on has fire retardant chemicals, and the clothes they wear have a variety of never press additives and fire retardants.

When children go to school, they are exposed to pesticides, insecticides, and herbicides along with other invisible chemicals. When they go to the dentist, they are given mercury amalgams to fill in the cavities. Day after day, we are exposed to indeterminable amounts of chemicals and toxins which build up in our bodies and can be stored in various places such as tissue, fat, and brain cells. With the increased amount of toxins, some working in a co-morbid manner, these poisons start to affect various organ and brain functions.

The rise of learning disabilities, autism, ADHD, anxiety, and depression are the results of the culmination of daily exposure to these harmful chemicals. The increase of children diagnosed with autism is just the tip of the iceberg of the increases of physical and mental disorders across the board.

These diagnoses are affecting every race, age group, and gender. Our bodies can no longer detox from the ongoing amount of chemicals to which we are exposed, and almost all health problems are on the rise.

It is hard for me to fathom the far reaching effects there will be over the coming 10, 20, 50 years. We are increasing the number of disabled people who cannot function on their own and will need extra services to live independently or stay home to live with their parents for the rest of their lives. We are producing generations of children that have numerous physical problems and mental impairments.

In this chapter, I will discuss the possible causes of autism and other disabilities that are plaguing our younger generations. Each can stand alone as having toxic effects, or they can combine together to debilitate the human body and mind. There can be a complex trial and error process to figure out what are the causes and what might be the solutions for treatment.

What Are Autism, Disabilities, and Diseases?

To begin, we need to acknowledge that there is a genetic/DNA type person who has a predisposition for autism, disabilities, and diseases. My discussion here is not a part of that genetic component.

If a child is born into this world healthy and then regresses into autism, there needs to be a strong consideration and search for types of cause(s) that have brought on the major change in the child's life. This book focuses on the possible causes to consider when your child has regressed to an autistic state.

First, what is the definition of autism? Autism spectrum disorder (ASD) and autism are both general terms for a group of complex disorders of brain development, physical problems, and disabilities. These disorders are characterized in varying degrees and by difficulties in social interaction, verbal and nonverbal communication, and repetitive behaviors. This explanation is from *Autism Speaks* and from the *DSM-5* (Diagnostic and Statistic Manual). ASD is usually diagnosed between the ages of 2 and 3 years old.

ASD affects over three million individuals in the U.S. and tens of millions worldwide. Autism is a wide-spectrum disorder, which means no two people with autism will have exactly the same symptoms. Government autism statistics suggest that prevalence rates have increased 10 to 17 percent annually in recent years.

Current data states that autism is affecting every 1 in 45 children, and one prediction says that by 2032, one in two children will suffer from some type of autism. That is astounding! If we do not make some radical medical and agricultural changes quickly, America and the world will be suffering from the biggest epidemic ever witnessed.

We now know that there is no one cause of autism, just as there is no one type of autism. It seems that there are two sides to the causes of ASD. One side states that the culprit is genetics or gene mutations; the other side believes that it is environmental factors influencing early brain development. I personally believe that it is more an environmental problem (approximately 90%) because of the information in the extensive research I have done.   Proof of the environmental damage is there for us to see, but it is rarely spoken about.

I believe that a great number of disabilities and diseases are created by environmental factors that were discussed earlier in this book.   I also surmise that there is no one cause, but a combination of factors affecting the vital parts of the body causing more and more health problems.

Consequently, these health complications increase the number of diagnoses of children with autism, learning disabilities, and a wide range of other disabilities and health issues which plague our schools and communities.   Eventually, these factor combinations progress into the diseases that are affecting older generations and the conditions from which they suffer.

The Vital Plan organization states that there are seven causes for disease:

1. Nutritional Stress - Poor quality of food and diet

2. Emotional Stress - The extremely fast paced change of the human condition and our inability to adjust to the stress

3. Toxins - (need I say more)

4. Physical Stress - Three types: trauma, temperature, and pressure

5. Free Radicals/Inflammation - The most significant factor in diseases and aging

6. Radiation - Radiation from gamma rays, x-rays, UV radiation, EMFs (electro-magnetic frequencies)

7. Microbes - Present in acute and chronic infections and diseases

Again, it certainly seems that we are bombarded with toxins, radiation, and microbes from every direction. If we do not have a healthy body to handle all of these factors, we become susceptible to infection and inflammation. The more that damage and free radicals build up in our bodies, the more susceptible we are to succumb to health problems, minor and major disabilities, and diseases.

We must change our perspective on living well and do everything possible to be as healthy as possible. We need to be healthy from a whole body standpoint with a "Body, Mind, and Spirit" point of view.   Life is supposed to be in balance, and the population as a whole is way out of balance.

A list of the commonly found characteristics identified among children and adults with ASD are as follows:

1. Lack of social skills

2. Lack of empathy (awareness of feelings of self and others)

3. No understanding of humor, irony, and sarcasm (takes things literally)

4. Dislike of physical and eye contact

5. Sensitivities to light, sound, smells, and taste

6. Speech and communicative problems or delays

7. Restricted repetitive behaviors

8. Physical tics and stimming (self-stimulating behaviors)

9. Obsessions

10. Low emotional and behavioral control

These characteristics or symptoms will range from mild to critical depending on the levels of toxins effecting the brain and body. Again, the ASD person can have one, two, or all the symptoms shown above. ASD can also range from highly functioning to severely nonfunctional. The more severely the symptoms are exhibited, the more extreme the diagnosis and problems are. That is the reason why they use the term "spectrum."

Facts and Statistics

Millions of children from the United States live with one or many diagnosed chronic illnesses. The *Academic Pediatrics* in 2011 estimated that 54% of children have at least one chronic illness. Here are just a few statistics from the Epidemic Answers organization:

Physical Illnesses

- Asthma - At least 1 in 8 non-African American children and approximately 1 in 6 African American children

- Allergic Eczema - 1 in 5 children

- Hay Fever (seasonal allergies) - 2 to 3 out of 5 children

- Food Allergies - 1 in 12 children under the age of 4 years old and 1 in 3 children have food intolerances.

- Celiac Disease - 1 in 80 children

- Obesity - 1 in 7 children

Millions of American children struggle with what were once termed "psychiatric" disorders, such as mood disorders, developmental delays, and learning disabilities.

Psychiatric Disorders (or a combination of physical and psychiatric)

- Autism - 1 in 45 children

- ADHD - 1 in 10 children

- Learning Disabilities - 1 in 6 children

- Severe Mood Dysregulation - (e.g. bipolar) 1 in 30 children

- Dyspraxia (impaired coordination and motor skills) - 1 in 10 children

- Pediatric depression - 1 in 30 children

- Obsessive Compulsive Disorder - 1 in 100 children

There are millions of children with undiagnosed chronic illnesses.

Here are some other interesting facts and statistics:

- About 1% of the world's population now has autism.

- More than 3.5 million Americans are diagnosed with ASD.

- The prevalence of autism in the U.S. has increased 119.4 percent since 2000.

- Autism services cost U.S. citizens $236-262 billion annually.

- It cost more than $8,600 extra per year to educate a student with autism.

The percentages of children with disabilities served under the IDEA are as follows:

- Specific Learning Disability - 35%

- Speech and Language Impairment - 21%

- Other Health Impaired - 12%

- Autism - 8%

- Intellectual Disability - 7%

- Developmental Delay - 6%

- Emotional Disturbance - 6%

- Multiple Disabilities - 2%

- Hearing Impairment - 1%

- Orthopedic Impairment - 1%

These statics are covering all races and ethnicities with only minor differences.

EPIDEMICS ARE NOT GENETIC.

The Effects on Our Immune System

To reiterate, I am not a medical doctor, and my comments in this section are strictly from research gathered from studies and experience outside of the "medical profession."

As stated previously, our bodies are being bombarded with toxins from every direction. Our immune system is complex and highly developed, comprised of a network of cells, tissues, and organs that work together to defend the body against attacks by "foreign" invaders.

Our skin is our first line of defense to keep the invaders out. Once toxins enter the body, our immune system will send out white blood cells to search out and destroy them. These invaders are primary microbes which are tiny organisms, such as bacteria, parasites, tumors, and fungi that cause infections. Viruses also cause infections but are too primitive to be classified as living organisms.

When the immune system hits the wrong target, however, it can unleash a torrent of disorders, including allergic diseases, arthritis, and a form of diabetes. If the immune system is crippled, other kinds of diseases result.

The immune system is generally divided into two parts. The first part constitutes the defenses with which you are born. These form what are known as the innate system. The second part of your immune system, known as immunity, develops as you grow.

Your immunity gives you protection against specific pathogens. Not only can this system recognize particular pathogens, but it also has a memory of this recognition, which means that if you encounter a certain pathogen twice, your immune system recognizes it the second time around. Your body will then respond more quickly to fight off the infection.

Since our bodies are exposed to so many and ever growing numbers of toxins in today's world, our immune system has to fight off more and more outside invaders. With the increase in the amount of toxins, our immune systems are overloaded and cannot keep up with the never ending bombardment.

There is a point where the immune system can't keep up with the demand on it, and various parts of the body start to show either disease or dysfunction. Various symptoms start to show up on a wide scale of mild to extreme. I believe that is why autism is called "The Autism Spectrum," because it covers a wide range of symptoms and effects and also includes different levels of dysfunction with another wide range of body and brain functions.

It Starts With Oxidative Stress and Inflammation

Many variables associated with living in modern industrial society seem to be working in concert to weaken our children's immune systems. From near the point of conception, the fetus is being exposed to toxics within the mother. The transfer of approximately 270 toxins has been discovered to go from mother to baby in the umbilical cord at birth.

Within hours after birth, doctors begin the onslaught of vaccines to the newborn baby. If the child is not breastfed, infant formulas expose them to a questionably healthy food source.

Month after month, year after year, the toxicity build up continues, and both physical and sometimes mental problems begin to be apparent. It is a perfect storm of genetic, epigenetic, and environmental factors that affects each child differently. Our children, the most vulnerable among us, are showing the earliest signs of this impact.

What is oxidative stress? Oxidative stress is essentially an imbalance between the production of free radicals and the ability of the body to counteract or detoxify their harmful effects through neutralization by antioxidants.

What is a free radical? A free radical is an oxygen containing molecule that has one or more unpaired electrons, making it highly reactive with other molecules and causing harm. Free radicals are created by eating too many calories and sugars, exposure to air pollution, and excessive stress.

What are antioxidants? Every cell that utilizes enzymes and oxygen to perform functions is exposed to oxygen free radicals that have the potential to cause serious damage to the cell. Antioxidants are molecules present in cells that prevent these reactions by donating an electron to the free radicals without becoming destabilized themselves.

An imbalance between oxidants and antioxidants is the underlying basis of oxidative stress which then leads to many pathophysiological conditions in the body. Some of these include neurodegenerative diseases, such as Parkinson's and Alzheimer's, gene mutations and cancers, chronic fatigue syndrome, fragile X syndrome, heart and blood vessel disorders, atherosclerosis, heart failure, heart attack, and inflammatory diseases. The list of diseases that are caused by oxidative stress is extensive.

What is inflammation? Inflammation is a localized protective response elicited by injury or destruction of tissues, which serves to destroy, dilute, or wall off both the injurious agent and the injured tissue. The inflammation response can be provoked by physical, chemical, and biological agents, including mechanical trauma, exposure to excessive amounts of sunlight, x-rays, radioactive materials, corrosive chemicals, extremes of heat and cold, or by infectious agents such as bacteria, viruses, and other pathogenic microorganisms.

Oxidative stress and inflammation are at the root cause of most health problems, diseases, and even autism. There are now a number of articles and books written about this connection between oxidative stress, inflammation, and autism. These causes can affect every organ and cell in the body. The brain and our digestive systems seem to exhibit the biggest connection to autism and the other problems surrounding their dysfunction. Inflammation could be the main cause of cancer.

In today's world, we are filled toxic substances which at some point create oxidative stress in the body, and the body reacts with inflammation. Without the proper detoxification and treatment to reduce stress and inflammation, this pattern happens day after day and increases the damage to body organs and cells.

At a certain point or after critical over-exposure to toxins, symptoms start to show up with various health and behavioral problems persisting. We can easily deduct from current statistics showing the rise in most diseases and other health problems that we are doing something wrong with our bodies and living the wrong lifestyles.

(2)

Comorbid Conditions

Autism is a broad term for a good reason. There is no one cause for the symptoms of autism, and there is no one solution for any attempts to treat, improve, or possibly "cure" it or its symptoms. The causes of autism, as well as the treatments and possible solutions, can be and usually are very complex.

Comorbidity is "the presence of one or more additional disorders (or diseases) co-occurring with a primary disease or disorder; the additional disorder may also be a behavioral or mental disorder." Autism falls under this spectrum. These comorbid conditions create a dynamic of great complexity.

The epidemic rates on the increases in numbers in children with the diagnosis of autism, ADHD, and other disabilities are a new phenomenon over just the last 20 years. This increase has caught every related profession by surprise, so we do not have all the answers or solutions. We are continually learning about autism, its causes, successful treatments, and which ones are treating only the symptoms but not the disease itself.

I strongly believe that individual doctors, therapists, and parents are finding some successful treatments; whereas our government agencies and bureaucratic systems (like the medical and educational fields) are moving at a snail's pace. We do not have the leisure to look at these disabilities with a fine toothed comb, dragging out analysis for years to get government approval, to put in place possible workable treatments and solutions.

There is an estimate that by 2032, 1 out of every 2 children will be affected by some type of autism or learning disability. If we (as a country and as individuals) do not approach this problem with every effort possible, we will be too late to save the ever increasing numbers of children injured by its magnitude. It is glaring at us! We all must act quickly to stop this epidemic which I refer to as "The Toxic Generations."

Children with autism have a much higher than expected rate to have all of the medical conditions studied, including eczema, allergies, asthma, ear and respiratory infections, gastrointestinal problems, severe headaches, migraines, and seizures. The death and mortality rates for autistic children and adults are three to ten times higher than the general population. One study found that deaths from gastrointestinal and respiratory disorders were 40 times higher than typical peers.

Impairments in communication and social interaction, by definition core symptoms of ASD, are higher. Autistic behaviors, including anxiety, aggression, agitation, irritability, impulsivity, lack of focus, sleep problems, self-stimulating, self-harming, and sensory difficulties, are also a part of the comorbid conditions. The cost in human toll and monetary drains on our current economy is incalculable.

It is very important to remember that, in most cases, there is not just one potential source; there are multiple agents affecting the child's body, mind, and functionality.

Very little research has been done on comorbid conditions, because the medical industry is only just starting to grasp the possible "most obvious" causes for autism. There is very little thought about combining comorbid conditions with the various other reasons for symptoms and disfunction.

My theory:

- Every child has a genetic blueprint from both sides of the parents from generations past. Include the blueprint of the prenatal mother's exposure to toxins and possible diseases.

- Every child's health can range from excellent to poor. So, their general health has a predisposition to what might lie ahead in the future. Parallel to this predisposition is the status of the child's immune system and how well prepared it is for the onslaught of germs, viruses, etc.

- Newborns will be exposed to vast amounts of toxins soon after birth, such as vaccines, environmental toxins, heavy metals, air and water pollutions, plastics, EMFs and poor quality food sources. The child's immune system and susceptibility to different toxins and conditions will determine the level of effect of these conditions and exposures.

- These exposures hit the immune system and, if overloaded, the body and mind start to develop symptoms and disfunction from mild to severe.

- The physical responses can be a combination of the following: auto immune system problems, various gut problems, candida, Lyme disease, biofilms, dermatological problems, allergies, chemical sensitivities, and food sensitivities.

- The mental responses can be a combination of the following: seizures, brain inflammation, communication deficits, cognitive impairments, ADHD symptoms, behavior and learning problems, anxiety and depression, sleep problems, sound and light sensory issues, and social problems.

- IMPORTANT: These responses can be in various combinations and severity.

At present, it is very difficult to analyze and decipher the medical conditions from which ASD children suffer and the appropriate treatments that will and can be effective to resolve the issues. The older the child gets, the less chance there is of experiencing reversible effects.

Mitochondrial Dysfunction

There is a connection between autism and the mitochondrial system. Because, toxins damage the body in ways we have discussed herein, they also damage this important system which literally creates the energy we have to live.

Mitochondria are tiny structures located within nearly all cells of the body. They create energy by generating adenosine triphosphate (ATP) which is the essential fuel that makes all of the body's functions possible. They are called the powerhouse of the cell. These structures are microscopic in size, and there are thousands per cell. Mitochondria are essential to life, and when they are damaged or functioning improperly, there can be negative effects on our balance of living and feeling well.

Listed below are some of the signs and symptoms of mitochondrial dysfunction, and notice how closely they resemble a variety of childhood disabilities, the very same disabilities we find in autism. This list is from an article by the non-profit organization Talk About Curing Autism (TACA).

- Developmental delay or regression

- Language impairment

- Social impairment

- Intellectual disability

- Neuropsychiatric symptoms (ADHD, anxiety, OCD, depression

- Seizures

- Headaches

- Hearing impairment

- Weakness

- Small stature

- Fatigue

- Gastrointestinal symptoms

- Endocrine disturbance

Current research suggests that mitochondrial dysfunction may be extremely important in these health conditions:

• Autism

• Bipolar Disease

• Schizophrenia

• Depression

• Diabetes

• Parkinson's disease

• Asthma

• Chronic fatigue syndrome

• Alzheimer's disease

Many different types of triggers can lead to mitochondrial dysfunction, and these may be either genetic, environmental, or a combination of both. Some triggers may be gene mutation, shortages of key vitamins or minerals, chemicals, heavy metal, drugs, certain bacteria or viruses, and stress.

This knowledge is an important breakthrough, but preventative steps are needed to eliminate the dysfunction and its results. Much more research is essential to understand this important aspect of the body's functions in order to prevent the new epidemic of childhood disabilities and diseases.

A study completed by University of California Davis concludes that children with autism experience deficits in a type of immune cell that protects the body from infection. The study concludes that the mitochondria of children with autism consume far less oxygen than typical children. Consequently, there is more oxidative stress which is a sign of decreased mitochondrial function.

Another study examined the use of Roundup/glyphosate on our food supply and deducted that its use can negatively affect mitochondrial function. In fact, the use of Roundup in agricultural parts of America connects to more prevalence of obesity in humans when you overlap the agricultural and obesity maps in America.

Chapter 3

Other Possible Effects of Toxic Exposure

(3)

Prenatal and In-Utero Effects

For couples trying to conceive, I highly recommend that both parents do extensive research and take steps necessary to detoxify their bodies and make certain life style changes prior to conception. It is critical to create a healthy environment for the new child to be in and out of the womb.

We are all toxic to a degree. New parents especially need to be as toxin free as possible and living a healthy lifestyle. Take an inventory of your home and work environments and remove all harmful substances. This may seem aggressive, but I feel the mother would be wise to not only consider replacing all dental amalgam's to get rid of mercury exposure but also to stop some current medications (that are not essential).

The brain of a fetus is the most vulnerable part of its body and is especially tender to exposure to toxins. The fetal brain begins growing in the 4th week of pregnancy at a rate of over 4,000 cells per second. Unlike an adult, the fetus does not have a functional blood brain barrier to protect itself from chemicals and neurotoxins. This lack of natural defense allows substances into the fetal brain with the potential to cause serious harm and disruption to the delicate brain growth process. The results could disrupt the brain, causing autism, ADHD, learning disabilities, and other childhood disorders.

There is more and more research showing the relationship of the mother's exposure to toxicities and the transfer of some of these to the embryo and fetus due to the blood to blood connections. If everything runs smoothly during the pregnancy, a midwife or doula birth can be considered to make sure the fetus's entry into the real world has as little trauma as possible.

Naturopathic advocates are increasing and advising to stay away from C-sections and induced labor which can harm the baby. All of these steps may not prevent autism and other problems, but they can at least give parents much better odds to have a healthy and thriving baby(s).

(3)

Birth Defects

This book will not address genetic birth defects, a small percentage of the total births that occur across our planet. My intention is to inform the reader of the environmental toxins which are creating many more birth defects than we are being told by federal agencies and media.

Every year, industrial facilities across the United States release more than 20 BILLION pounds of toxic substances known to cause birth defects, developmental delays, and other neurological problems in children. Also, as many as four million potentially toxic chemical mixtures can be found in homes and businesses around the country. Some homes and businesses might not have been tested for safety.

Birth defects from toxins can occur when a pregnant woman inhales, ingests, or otherwise absorbs toxic chemicals or substances into her body. Even though such congenital abnormalities are potentially preventable, thousands of children are born every year with birth defects from toxins.

The most common substances are lead, mercury, arsenic, cadmium, pesticides, organic solvents, and toxic household chemicals. Even chlorinated drinking water poses a risk of anomalies during pregnancy. Prescription drugs and over-the-counter drugs also have risks for birth defects.

The "Autism Spectrum Disorders Report" from the *National Birth Defects Registry* states that children with autism have a higher chance of having some other type of birth defect condition(s) along with their diagnosis of autism. They reported that the most frequent birth defects that coincide with autism are craniofacial, central nervous system (CNS), limb, syndromes, gastrointestinal, genitourinary, heart, chromosome, and growth.

(3)

Possible Causes of Autism and Comorbid Combinations

There is no one cause for autism. Autism is a complex array of health problems that have been created by comorbid conditions (see Comorbid Conditions in Chapter 2) due to numerous possible factors. After reading many books and articles on the potential causes of autism, I found information focused only on *one* particular cause or another. Herein I will examine autism from a broader point of view.

Based on my findings, I constructed a theory which I believe has validity and will shed a new light on what is happening to the young and old of our country and around the world. My deductions are not scientifically proven and I am not a medical doctor, but I believe these conclusions have merit.

We all have genes and DNA passed down to us from our parents. At conception, both the mother's and father's physical predispositions, along with genetic faults and weaknesses, can be important to the well-being of the newborn child. If the parents have a weakness or a predisposition to a specific disease or defect, the chances of it being passed down are high. Without specifics or percentages, just consider what some of the same traits, physical symptoms, or diseases your parents passed down to you.

Toxins in the mother's body are transferred to the unborn child through the blood from the placenta in the uterus. If the mother is exposed to any chemicals or toxins during pregnancy, the fetus will have some transfer to its body. We need to consider the types and quantities of chemicals and/or toxins in the exposure and the amount and duration of exposure. In addition, there are comorbid conditions and/or reactions that combine to determine the child's condition.

When a child is born, there is susceptibility to other types of exposure to chemicals and toxins in the new environment. If we add vaccines, air and water pollutions, and various other toxins mentioned herein, the child's immune system will continue to weaken. There seems to be a point where the natural detoxification process can no longer keep up, and the child becomes toxic. Various symptoms start to show up. Remember, each baby is different, and their predisposition to exposures, quality of their immune system, and ability to detoxify play a major role as to whether or not the child will have health problems (i.e. autism, disabilities, diseases, other health issues, etc. The symptoms can be mild to severe and can be in comorbid combinations.

Following are some possible results from toxic exposures:

1) Immune system: Our immune system is extremely valuable to our body. It protects us from invaders, both interior and exterior, and will react to fight off these invaders for basic self-preservation. Presently, researchers are exploring whether changes within the developing immune system could compromise nervous system development and ultimately lead to such disorders as autism ADHD, and other diseases and disabilities. I believe there is a domino effect on body organs and systems; as various toxins disrupt them, they start to degrade and function poorly, which results in more symptoms and problems. This pattern continues until the body is disrupted enough to consider the resulting condition a disorder or disability. As the immune system starts to function improperly, inflammation begins and persists for a long period of time; i.e., the more inflammation created (beginning in the womb), the more severe the problems become.

2) Vaccines: I know that use of vaccines and their connections to autism is a very controversial topic. I investigated thimerosal's (a mercury-based preservative) relation to autism over 15 years ago. If you believe what the government and pharmaceutical manufacturers say, thimerosal has been taken out of the MMR vaccines and is found only in flu shots. Beyond thimerosal, the problem surrounding the use of vaccines is the quantity and the combination of vaccines in shots given at various times throughout childhood and adult years. The number of vaccines that are required by schools and government adds up to over 60 vaccines over the course of a person's life. This amount has tripled in the last 40 years. Even though the use of thimerosal has supposedly been eliminated, I strongly believe that a high percentage of young children are still vulnerable to vaccines and the large volume being currently used and required.

3) Gut Issues: The first signs of health difficulties usually show up in the gut/intestinal system. The problems can range from minor to severe. Much research has suggested that that the digestive system is the body's second brain. Every indication points to a direct connection

between the gut and brain, and if you treat the gut, other problems will become resolved.

4) Candida: Candida is a yeast that is supposed to exist in small amounts among much greater amounts of friendly bacteria in the intestinal flora. Unfortunately, in this age of antibiotics, medications, chlorinated water, and chemicals in our foods, all of which destroy the friendly bacteria, the Candida yeast is left intact. Candida overgrows in the intestinal tract, filling up the space left by the friendly bacteria that have died. Candida thrives on refined sugars and processed foods. It is associated with poor digestion, hence, poor nutritional intake, because the intestines can't absorb the necessary vitamins and minerals from food and digestion.

5) Lyme disease: Lyme disease is one of the fastest growing infectious diseases in the nation. The disease is caused by the bite of a tick infected with Borrelia Burgdorferi and may be complicated by other parasites or co-infections. Lyme disease can have long term deadly effects over time. Again, if a child's immune system is compromised, any contact with this infection can only multiply the physical symptoms of their autistic tendencies.

6) Pyroluria: Pyroluria is a common metabolic condition that occurs when Pyrrole, a key component of hemoglobin, is overproduced by the liver and not fully excreted in the urine. Pyroluria creates an imbalance and a deficiency in zinc, manganese, and other B vitamins. This shortage affects the functioning of your entire body and mind, including immune system, digestion, cognitive functioning, and emotions.

7) Biofilms: Biofilms are formed in the blood. They are built by bacteria which group together and weave a protective web or matrix about them in order to protect them from the immune system. So, the bacteria remain alive, fermenting, metabolizing, and sending their toxins into the blood stream.

8) Viruses: Viruses are always found in autistic children. The majority of autistic children have chronic viral infections. Anytime the immune system is wiped out by chronic Candida or Lyme infections, children are susceptible to developing chronic viral infections. Sometimes these viruses can reside in the brain in the myelin sheath.

9) Over-use of antibiotics: In our current world, many doctors give out prescriptions for antibiotics like candy. When you have a child with a compromised immune system, the over-use of antibiotics leaves many children with no "good" bacteria. Then they are vulnerable to other invaders of all sorts. An autistic child may be sick or ill fairly often. Antibiotic use can multiply the effects of other dysfunctions in the body and might lead to more severe symptoms.

10) EMFs, cell phones, and wireless technologies: Electromagnetic frequencies surround us. The increased use of wireless technologies gives us a constant barrage of frequencies that we cannot touch, see, or feel - but are there! EMF exposure increases the production of toxic microbes and endotoxins. The primary sources of EMFs are the following:

- Electric fields from anything that has voltage; electrical wiring, lights, appliances, and outlets

- Magnetic fields, the major source being next to your electric meter by your house

- Power Lines, either above or below ground

- Metal plumbing - Older metal plumbing pipes can carry a current.

- Wireless communication - Cell phones, cell towers, routers, and cordless phones

Humans are no longer healthy, especially the younger generations. They have been exposed to many more toxic substances during their lives than older generations. Just one of these possible exposures does not necessarily create health problems, but when there are combinations, the possibility of effects is multiplied.

The problem with diagnosing and treating autism and other disorders lies in the possible combinations of causes, and they are very hard to figure out. Basically, autism is a new disease of our time, and we are just starting to scratch the surface to understand it. Doctors or clinicians need to figure out the percentages of each possible toxic exposure which is affecting the child. Each child is different, and all the percentages will be different also. It is almost like spinning a roulette wheel and guessing on a number.

(3)

Nerve and Brain Damage

Toxins have a wide range of effects on our environment and our bodies. These effects can be very mild and subtle to extreme and drastic. There does seem to be a parallel between the amount of toxic exposure and the severity of autism. Science has not been able to figure out the sensitivities and the tolerances of the human body, which are so individualized, and how and why some people are affected more or less than others who have the exact same amount of exposure.

Nerve damage can be caused by exposure to a variety of neurotoxins. Neurotoxins alter the normal activity of the nervous system in a way to cause damage to the nervous tissue, brain cells, and brain function. They can eventually disrupt and damage nerve cells depending on the amount of exposure and duration. Symptoms of exposure can appear immediately or may be delayed. The symptoms may include limb weakness or numbness, loss of memory, vision and/or intellect, uncontrollable obsessive and compulsive behaviors, delusions, headaches, cognitive and behavioral problems, and sexual dysfunction. Some individuals may be more vulnerable than others.

Some common neurotoxins are as follows: acetone, acetylene, aflatoxins, albuterol, aluminum, ammonia, atrazine, benzene, butane, caffeine, captopril, cocaine, codeine phosphate, deionized water, diazepam, digoxin, ethanol, fluoxetine, gasoline vapors, kerosene, lead, and mercury. These and other chemicals are responsible for widespread behavioral and cognitive problems. Dr. David Bellinger determined Americans have collectively forfeited forty-one million IQ points because of neurotoxin exposure and damage!

Our society is being given gross misinformation about the dangers of neurotoxins. I believe that neurotoxins are affecting each and every individual, young, old, small, and large. We are living in a sea of toxins, and to some degree, we basically can't get out of the pool to reduce our exposure. We can't easily determine who is over-sensitive to these exposures and who can resist and detoxify. Determination is individual by individual.

Autism to Alzheimer's -

Toxic Effects From Young to Old

I think that the connection of autism to toxicity is well known, especially the exposure to mercury. Also, as the diagnoses of autism started to rise over the past 20 to 30 years, there has been a massive explosion in Alzheimer's disease and other forms of dementia paralleling this increase. During this time frame, the advent of "mysterious" disorders and syndromes such as chronic fatigue, fibromyalgia, and autoimmune diseases have also increased.

A shocking statistic reveals that over half the population in the developed world will currently end their days with Alzheimer's disease if they live to be 85 or older. More than four million Americans now have Alzheimer's disease, which should place it in the epidemic category. Individuals suffering with Alzheimer's and autism show striking similarities, with the exception that they are on different ends of a lifespan. Some say that there are over 160 likenesses between the two. Here are some that have more than obvious parallels in both conditions:

- A major impact on memory and recognition of faces and voices

- Loss of energy, lethargy, and passivity

- Loss of intellect and concentration

- Sensory overload, withdrawal from social contact, and poor eye contact

- Catatonic state and emotionless expressions

- Little, if any, conception of time and space

- Anxiety, depression, mood swings, and aggression

- Digestive system problems

- Insomnia and sleep problems

The damage and effects of mercury poisoning are very similar, if not exactly the same. Alzheimer's disease was first described in 1906, just a few decades after the widespread use of amalgam fillings. Studies showed that Alzheimer sufferers have two to three times the brain mercury levels than people without the disease. There are just too many parallels between the two to disregard the similarities and possible effects of mercury toxicity in the brain. Other chemicals and pesticides that could contribute to both autism and Alzheimer's are aluminum, pesticides, and DDT (a banned pesticide).

Chapter 4

Where do we go from here?

For the past 20 years I have witnessed the dramatic rise in numbers of students that qualify for special education services and seen the severity of disabilities increase. In 1996, it seemed we had only one or two children in a given school who had the diagnosis of autism. This year in 2017, in the high school to which I was assigned, the total number of children with the label of autism is closer to 50!

Yes, we are diagnosing more autistic children and the severity of their disabilities is getting far more harsh. I believe that we are at **epidemic** levels, and if we, as a country, society, and community do not react and make the changes necessary to stop our children from getting these debilitating diagnoses, our country cannot survive as we know it. The United States will undergo severe changes and repercussions with the cost of caring for these children due to long term placement and other types of treatments. Also, many of these individuals will not be able to contribute to society, pay taxes, and propagate future generations.

Today, the treatments that are approved by our government and medical institutions are composed of pharmaceutical drugs or a few "scientifically proven" practices or theories which have their place but also have limitations. We need to prevent the increases of children with disabilities, and we need to treat the current and future children better. As the parent of a child with disabilities, your role has drastically changed with the upsurge of children diagnosed with autism and other diseases in the 21st century. You have had to educate yourself on information that has normally been left up to the doctor. You as a parent have had to learn to be a therapist, nutritionist, and be medically aware of your child's conditions, sensitivities, and triggers.

This chapter is totally dedicated to alternative non-invasive treatment options and steps you must consider to improve the health of your child. I cannot recommend which one you should choose or try. But my objective is for you to realize that there are many more treatment options that are not harmful to your child!

You need to have an open mind, do your research, and consider if these non-invasive treatments will be helpful to your child. Then go out to your community to find who may offer these treatments. Please realize that every child has individual needs, and what might work for one might not work for another. The reality is there is a vast system of people discovering a variety of different treatments which are not known to most peoplle; there is a new revolution in health, healing, and ways of treating disabilities.

I strongly believe that in America we have been increasingly exposed to toxins for the past 60 to 70 years. The effects of this exposure are now generational as the parents pass down these toxins to their children who pass them down to their children. In the past 20 years especially, toxic exposure of nearly every kind has multiplied dramatically. These toxins and chemicals have saturated our water, food, and air.

Again, 77,000 chemicals are produced in the United States alone. Over 3,000 chemicals have been added to our food supply. Over 10,000 chemical solvents, emulsifiers, and preservatives are used in food processing. Most Americans have between 400-800 chemicals stored in their bodies, typically in their fat cells. So what do you do about the children?

The first step is to determine which toxins are prevalent in the child's body. If your child's disabilities are severe, your pediatrician should do the appropriate tests to make this determination. If the symptoms are less severe, you could consider doing the testing yourself through lab work or hair analysis. After you know what toxins are in your child's body, then you must decide on a detoxification plan to rid the body of the harmful toxins.

(4)
Biomedical Interventions

If you are going to a standard pediatrician or doctor and are not happy with your services, I recommend you make an appointment with a doctor that specializes in child disabilities or MAPS doctor. MAPS stands for Medical Academy of Pediatric Special Needs, and these doctors have completed a medical program specializing in children with disabling conditions. As of 2017, there are only a few hundred MAPS doctors, so they might not be available to you and your child.

What is the Biomedical Intervention model? It is an individualized treatment protocol looking at all the possible symptoms and comorbid conditions from which the child is suffering. It usually starts with a thorough medical history with an extensive blood workup and physical exam. The blood workup will detect any toxic and heavy metals build up in the body and brain.

A treatment plan is developed by the determination of what is wrong and what is needed to attack these conditions. Some of the areas of examination are: gastrointestinal issues, mitochondrial dysfunction, vitamin and mineral deficiencies, neurological disorders, and any other symptoms the child might be exhibiting. Treatments could include dietary interventions, allergy treatments, vitamins, mineral and supplement regimens, and detoxification programs.

Most children on the spectrum have various symptoms of gastrointestinal problems which include:

- diarrhea, constipation, reflux, food cravings, bloating, fatigue, aggression, sleep difficulties, spaciness, agitation, inappropriate behaviors, and stimming (self-stimulatory behaviors).

The possible causes of the gastrointestinal problems may be due to one or more of the following:

- bacteria, yeast, or fungus overgrowth, leaky gut syndrome, unbalanced intestinal flora, overuse of antibiotics, and inflammation.

Children on the spectrum have a tendency to have impaired immune systems and show symptoms like fevers, compulsive behaviors, eczema, and aggression. Immune system dysfunctions can also impact the brain development and/or brain function and can lead to viruses, leaky gut, predisposition to autoimmune diseases, and other sensitivities.

Children that have toxic levels of materials in their bodies will exhibit some of the following:

- sensory issues, sleep difficulties, stimming, impulsivity, aggression, compulsiveness, night sweats, anxiety, and lack of speech.

Detoxification abnormalities in the body contribute to the buildup of heavy metals in tissues including the brain.

The most common treatments used are gluten free/casein free diets, allergy testing, probiotics, and digestive enzymes. An appropriate detoxification plan will depend on the toxin problems at hand.

(4)

Detox...Detox...and stay Detoxed!

The information provided here is to give you choices, not to diagnose or give you direct or indirect medical advice. Please consult your physician before making any medical decisions about you or your children.

In all the articles and books I read on detoxification of the human body, the website and testing site *Doctor's Data* seems to explain it best. Elements are the building blocks of all chemical compounds, and human exposure to them occurs both from natural and anthropogenic sources. Many elements are considered nutrients and are essential for proper functioning of the body. These are generally divided between macro minerals such as calcium, magnesium, potassium, sodium, and zinc, and trace minerals including selenium, iodine, boron, and molybdenum.

Conversely, there are a number of elements that are toxic to the human body, interfere with its functioning, and undermine health, such as mercury, lead, cadmium, aluminum, and arsenic. These toxic metals have no known physiological functions. They can be toxic to organ systems and may disrupt the balance of essential nutrients. Toxic metals and essential element status can be assessed in urine, blood, feces, and hair.

If you believe that you and/or your child have some sort of toxins in your body, please consult your doctor and consider taking the following tests:

- A comprehensive blood elements test will assess the status of key elements and electrolytes. This assessment will determine if you are depleted in certain elements or have specific toxins in your body.

- A urine toxic and essential elements test is used to evaluate exposure to potentially toxic elements and wasting of nutrient elements.

- A creatinine clearance is a test for estimating glomerular filtration rate and renal function.

- Hair elements is an assessment which provides information regarding recent and ongoing exposure to toxic metals, especially methylmercury and arsenic.

- The fecal test provides direct indications of diet exposure to toxic metals and potential for toxic metal burden.

- Other recommended tests in the research were IgF food allergy, organic acid test, metabolic screening, heavy metals assessment via stool, blood, urine and hair, glutathione assessment, amino acids, liver enzymes and kidney function, vitamin A and D, comprehensive digestive stool analysis, complete blood count, urinary peptides, methylmalonic acids (MMA), serum B12, ferritin and iron levels, thyroid function, plasma, zinc, cholesterol, and fatty acids.

How do you detox (remove toxic materials from) your body? It will depend on what toxins you have in your body and what are the best ways to rid your body of them? There are multitudes of products and programs that specialize in detoxing your body. You will need to match the toxin to the type of detoxification needed. Here are the most common types of detoxifications to consider:

- Colon cleanse

- Liver and kidney cleanse

- Parasite cleanse

- Candida cleanse

- Toxic metal cleanse (chelation)

- Glutathione supplement

If you do your research on the internet, you can find many programs and detox supplement manufacturers. Listed below are some at home detox regimens that you can do on your own:

- Raw/alkaline foods

- Juice fasting

- Cleansing spices

- Exercising, sweating, and saunas

- Fasting

- Magnesium Chloride (Epsom salt baths)

- Detox Clay

- Water flushes

- Coffee enemas

- Foods that detoxify

- Ion Cleanse foot bath: At the last TACA NOW convention in October 2017, I was introduced to A Major Difference, Inc. AMD has been manufacturing the IonCleanse total body detoxification and relaxation system since 2002. The IonCleanse by AMD helps the body detox through the healing power of ions, because their powerful charge cleanses the body more effectively than any other method of detox. The process is safe, relaxing, and non-invasive with no harmful side effects. AMD's patented technology creates both positively and negatively charged ions.   Thus, you can address toxicity at all levels within the body. AMD cannot make any medical claims, but they offer an unprecedented 60-day, 100% money-back guarantee on the system.   In 2016, the "Thinking Mom's Revolution Study" by AMD showed the results of the Autism Treatment Evaluation Checklist (ATEC) for a large number of ASD children. Their scores improved over a period of 30 days, 60 days, 90 days, and 120 days.   Overall average reduction (desired) in these scores was 55% over the 120-day period. Look at the "Featured products" section at the back of this book or go to *amajordifference.com/?utm_source=awc* for more information.

Please note that some children cannot and will not be able to do a number of these recommendations.

Some toxins are easily disposed of and others are not. Detoxification is a process that could take a period of time.   During this process, it is highly suggested that a good diet and life-style changes are integrated to assist with the body's transformation and rebalancing of you or your child's health. Detoxing the body is good for everyone.

(4)

Diet Choices

After World War II, the United States made a number of changes to agricultural and food production. Yes, the rise of "fast" foods and easy-to-make processed foods seemed to be a great idea then, because it cut down the time in making meals. But this change has come with a cost which not many expected or realized.

Small home grown family farms gradually transformed into corporate farming. The rise of the chemical companies' influence and the development of pesticides, herbicides, and insecticides usage on our food sources has poisoned the foods that we eat. The agricultural mission statement is to produce the most crops per acre possible without concern for the crops' nutritional value or safety of customers.

Americans have been forced into a health crisis that is affecting each and every one of us, especially this generation of children. We have to open our eyes and minds to realize what is being forced upon us without our consent or knowledge. We have filled our bodies with toxins that have created an "imbalance" in our health!

Our organs are struggling to be healthy. Our brains can no longer function well; there are rising neurological problems among all age groups. Yet our government agencies such as the FDA and the Department of Agriculture continue to let companies like Monsanto genetically modify our food sources for their profit.

As a population, we are just beginning to take back control of our health. The Organic Revolution is the result of people saying "NO" to GMOs and foods covered with pesticides, herbicides, and insecticides. Americans are looking for healthier alternatives than what is being sold in most grocery stores. But, we still need to research and determine which diets are necessary for children that have already been affected by the toxic exposures in our environment. We have growing numbers of children who have food sensitivities and food intolerances.

In the past 20 years, Americans have started to transform our diets because of the rise of autism, ADHD, anxiety and a plethora of other ailments from which children and adults are suffering. We have to change our thinking and realize "the food we eat, is our medicine." Parents need to become aware of their children's food sensitivities, actively test for toxins, and implement the diet that fits the best. A consultation with your doctor, nutritionist, or dietician is recommended. A list of the following diets from the organization Talk About Curing Autism (tacanow.org) are available for children with autism, ADHD, and some other disabilities - these have been proven to help improve general overall health and symptoms.

- GFCFSF (Gluten, Casein, Soy-free): This diet has been the most successful (91% positive reaction) for children with autism and can help with leaky gut.

- Whole Food Diet (Real Foods Diet): Eating as organic as possible and free of pesticides, etc.

- SCD (Specific Carbohydrate Diet): Designed for inflammatory bowel disease

- GAPS (Gut and Psychology Syndrome): Sugar and grain free

- LOD (Low Oxalate Diet): For improved kidney as well as mitochondria and glutathione function

- Body Ecology Diet: Similar to the GFCF diet

- Feingold Diet: Removing all artificial colors, flavors, and preservatives

- Weston Price Diet: The whole cooking diet with raw dairy

- Rotation Diet: Used to control food allergies by eating biologically related foods on the same day and then waiting four days before eating them again

- Element Diet: An eastern medical method using the basis of the five elements of fire, earth, metal, water, and wood

- Ketone Diet: Puts the body in a state of ketosis by eliminating all carbohydrates and sugar

Many children can be very picky eaters, and you might find resistance or rejection at first.

(4)
Herbs and Supplements

Any herbs or supplements need to be used with caution and care for the individual, especially children under the age of 18 years. The herbs listed can assist your efforts but cannot be considered a cure. Please do your own research and/or talk with a naturopathic doctor.

Mental Health and Function:

- Kava Kava, St. John's Wort, Valerian, Bacopa, Gensend, Holy Basil, Chamomile, Brahmi, Got Kola, Sage, Kudzu, and Catnip

Digestive and Urinary Systems:

- Licorice, Milk Thistle, Peppermint Oil, Ginger, Senna, Gentian, Uva Ursi, Aloe, Gamma Orizanol, Rose Hips, Anise, and Celery Seed

Pain and Inflammation:

- Arnica, Feverfew, Willow Bark, Devil's Claw, Chinese Skullcap, Marjoram, Thyme, Meadowsweet, Cat's Claw, Wood Betony, and Witch Hazel

This book is not intended to be a substitute for medical advice of a licensed physician. The reader should consult with their doctor in any matters relating to their health.

(4)

Homeopathic, Integrative, Ayurveda, and Other Remedies

Homeopathic Medicine: The American Institute of Health (AIH) describes Homeopathy as the practice of medicine that embraces a holistic and natural approach to the treatment of the sick. Homeopathy is holistic because it treats the person as a whole, rather than focusing on a diseased part or a labeled sickness. The guiding principle of Homeopathy is stated as "let likes cure likes."

Integrative Medicine: Integrative medicine is healing-oriented medicine that takes account of the whole person, including all aspects of lifestyle. It emphasizes the therapeutic relationship between practitioner and patient, is informed by evidence, and makes use of all appropriate therapies.

Ayurvedic Medicine: Ayurveda is one of the world's oldest holistic (whole body) healing systems. It was developed over 3000 years ago in India. It is based on the belief that health and wellness depend on a delicate balance between mind, body, and spirit. Its main goal is to promote good health, not fight disease. But treatments may be geared toward specific health problems.

These alternative forms of medicine are growing in popularity in the U.S. and are being used more and more on children with disabilities such as autism and ADHD. Since they look at the child as a "whole," the techniques used are non-toxic and much different than the western medicine approach.

So, when should you consider using these methods or options? If your child seems physically stable but still has a constant medical problem(s) that can't be solved, these "whole body" viewpoints might make the difference.

(4)
Other Possible Treatments

CEASE Therapy was developed by Dr. Tinus Smits and is a form of homeopathic medicine. "CEASE" stands for Complete Elimination of Autistic Spectrum Expression. Dr. Smits concludes that autism is an accumulation of different causes, and about 70% is due to vaccines, 25% to toxic medications and other toxic substances, and 5% to some diseases. CEASE therapists utilize Isotherapy, a treatment which uses causative substances (such as decreasing doses of vaccines) as a homeopathic remedy; their profound toxic effects can be witnessed as the children begin to react to the remedies. The problem is there are only about 100 Cease therapists across the country.

EMDR Therapy, short for Eye Movement Desensitization and Reprocessing, is a powerful new psychotherapy technique which has been very successful in helping people who suffer from trauma, anxiety, panic, and other emotional problems. It has recently being used with children with autism and ADHD. EMDR therapy uses bilateral stimulation, right/ left eye movement, or tactile stimulation, which repeatedly activates the opposite sides of the brain, releasing emotional experiences that are trapped in the nervous system.

(4)

NEWSFLASH!! Homeopathic Vaccines

I am against vaccinations because, as a school psychologist, I have witnessed the suffering of teens who have received these vaccinations. In 1986, Congress passed a bill allowing the pharmaceutical industry to be free from liablity for damages from vaccines in order to prevent lawsuits against them. That changed everything!

The number of required vaccines started rising from 8 per childhood in the 1950's to over 60 vaccines in 2017. Since the pharmaceutical companies were not liable, Congress had to set up a fund for parents to get financial help if their child had some type of damaging effects from the administering of vaccines. In other words, these companies are not held responsible for the damaging effects that they are creating in our society, and the government sets up a fund to pay for their mistakes. How can this have happened?

The U.S. spends the most on health care and has one of the highest child vaccination rates in the world. This country is crippled by a chronic disease and disability epidemic that costs more than $2 trillion annually. Just look at the statistics which speak for themselves. I do not know how America will be able to survive the costs of medical, housing, and supervision care of this ever expanding population of toxic children. Parents MUST do research and take responsibility for the lives of their children regarding government guidelines and doctor vaccine promotions.

If you choose to have your child vaccinated, please consider the following options:

- Ask your doctor for ingredients in the vaccines and if there are non- toxic alternatives.

- Space out the vaccines and avoid multiple vaccines at one time. Little bodies can't handle all those toxins in one dose.

- Consider homeopathic alternatives to vaccines.

(I live in California and checked with a district superinten- dent who said the California Department of Education would not accept the homeopathic alternative). Please check with your state to find out if this is an option for you and your child.

What is homeooprophylaxis (homeopathic vaccination)? It satisfies the process of naturally acquiring a disease by providing a tiny dose of the disease without any of the risks. The procedure uses remedies called nosodes. Nosodes are given orally, one disease at a time, to stimulate the general immunity of the body.

Homeopathic vaccine history goes back to the early 1800s and is considered a non-toxic alternative to standard vaccines. I highly recommend the book *The Solution,* by Kate Birch and Cilla Whatcott, if you are looking for alternatives to standard vaccinations. The new motto for the anti-vaccines is "Show us the science and give US a choice."

Electromagnetic Frequencies, Vibrational, And Subtle Healing Techniques

Believe it or not, we live in a world of electrons, photons, and electrical frequencies. Almost everything is emitting a frequency; some are barely detectable, but they are still transmitting. For most people, these frequencies cannot be detected by the senses, but they are proven to exist by certain scientific instruments. Many ancient healing techniques have been based on the fact that human body frequencies are "out of balance," causing pain, discomfort, illnesses, and even death. There are a variety of healing techniques for re-balancing frequencies in the body.

Since the advent of electricity, man has been experimenting and modifying electricity to somehow heal the body. Many scientists were innovators into our modern age of industrialism and convenience. Nicholas Tesla was one of the frontrunners in inventions using electricity, and many of his patents are among the ones used for healing.

Royal Rife deducted that all organs in the human body have a frequency and developed a machine that emitted frequencies to heal specific parts of the body's functioning organs and systems. Pulsating Electromagnetic Frequency (PEMF) machines have been steadily growing in use even though western medical organizations have not accepted these modes of treatment.

What is vibrational energy healing? Vibrational energy healing, or harmonic healing, dates back to ancient civilizations of the Chinese, Aztecs, and Egyptians. Vibrational medicine influences the body and energy field by changing its frequency using a variety of different modalities. The goal of vibrational healing is to activate the body's energies toward equilibrium and balance. Some of these different modalities are:

- homeopathic medicine.

- Chinese medicine, such as acupuncture, chakra healing

- herbal remedies.

- electromagnetic treatments.

- light, color, and sound healing.

- movement/exercise programs, such as Ti Chi, Qigong, yoga, and martial arts.

- hands-on methods, such as massage, acupressure, Reiki, Jim Shin Jujitsu.

- magnetics.

- kinesiology.

- distance healing.

- spiritual practices, such as prayer, mindfulness, meditation.

- subtle techniques, such as essential oils, gems, flower elixirs and essence, crystal and stone healing.

- Grounding techniques.

Everything you introduce into your mind, body, and energy field affects you to some degree. With positive intentions you can increase the effects of healthy vibrations in your everyday life. Some helpful tips that can increase vibrational techniques are:

- Regular exercise, healthy diet, and a good night's sleep.

- Use of superfoods and herbs.

- Creativity such as music, arts, and dance.

- Being aware of toxic foods, chemicals, negative emotions, and relationships.

What is the grounding technique? In today's world, the younger generation has been bombarded with computer, iPad, iPhone, and Wi-Fi/ EMF frequencies. Many children do not go outside and play in the grass or dirt; they play video games. This lack of outside play has led to a number of children not being grounded. Grounding technique is a set of simple strategies to help an individual get grounded with the earth. It helps them learn to be in the present and be aware of what is happening "now." It can help with the rampant growth of anxiety and depression and even PTSD. A few grounding techniques are:

- Deep breathing.

- Being aware of your surroundings.

- Going outside and sitting in the sun for 10 minutes.

- Walking bare foot in the grass or sitting under a tree.

- Feeling the emotions of being alive and being grateful for your life.

The use of vibrational healing methods are becoming more commonplace and accepted by our culture. As more people experience these various techniques, the more they will be used to assist us in dealing with the "stressed-out" world in which we live. Again, you must do your research and decide which technique resonates with you. There is no one solution and no one answer.

Light, Color, and Sound Therapies

We live in a world of frequencies. As strange as it seems, below the surface of our realities lie the frequency wave lengths of light, color, and sound. We can only see a fraction of what is all around us. The light that creates color is comprised of various wave frequencies, and the sounds that we hear have their own frequencies.

Light Therapy

Types of Light:

- The Sun: Without it the human race would not exist nor would life itself. The sun is our main source of light and heat. Since the Industrial Age, humans have been trying to duplicate the sun's attributes of shedding light where there is darkness and heat where there is cold. We succeeded with the first light bulb in the late 1800's and advanced from there.

- Full-spectrum white light: It is called full spectrum because its light covers the widest area of the visible spectrum of light. It also is the closest to the emissions of the sun.

- LED: Meaning "light-emitting diode," is a semi-conductor device that emits visible light when an electric current passes through it.

- Infrared: An LED light that also emits infrared energy along with the light

- Laser: The official definition is "Light Amplification by Stimulating Emission of Radiation" and is a device that amplifies light, then releases it in a coherent powerful beam. Only lasers are truly monochromatic and the band of width is very narrow.

- Monochromatic: Meaning "one color"

The use of light for healing goes back only to the early 1900's, since man-made light is a fairly recent invention. Due to advances in technology and the ability to manufacture better products, the use of LED, infrared, and lasers are becoming more accepted as treatment modalities for a variety of diseases and ailments. The use of these products for children with disabilities such as autism, ADHD, and other problems is on the rise.

Some of the beneficial uses of light therapy and treatment are as follows:

- Full-spectrum white light is most commonly called SAD light and is used for depression and other ailments that are related to "lack of sunlight" disorders or ailments.

- LED light therapy comes in a few colors and can be used for pain relief, promotes increase in circulation, and speeds up healing of wounds and sprains. It is beneficial to organs and boosts mitochondria function. The use of LED light has been used to balance the Chakras and is used with acupuncture to improve its benefits. Presently, LED light therapy is being used with children with autism, ADHD, traumatic brain injury, and other neurological disorders such as anxiety and depression.

- Laser therapy has been increasing in possible uses for a wide range of disabilities and illnesses. The use of lasers can stimulate the mitochondria, which in turn will produce more ATP (adenosine triphosphate) which generates energy within the body. It can lower inflammation, and decrease edema and excitotoxicity in the brain. Transcranial laser stimulation is being used for TBI (traumatic brain injury) and depression.

Color Therapy

The father of color therapy is Dinshah Ghadiali from India who started experimenting with various colors and their healing effects on the human body. Similar to other frequency theories, he deducted that certain colors were helpful for various ailments and also where to place the color on the body. Dinshah believed that ailments were related to bodily tasks being out of balance and that using color would rebalance the body's functions. The use of colors also corresponds with balancing the chakras.

Sound Therapy

Sound and its uses have been around for a long time. With the first grunts of communication and the first beating of makeshift drums, sound has been used therapeutically. Sound can be music to our ears, because it can change our moods and feelings and can make us dance and sing. Sound can motivate us; it is a multi-sensory experience; it is processed in both hemispheres of the brain; it is non-verbal; and it can make people bond together.

By itself, sound can stimulate or calm your mind. Many advancements in sound have been developed over the past 20 years with the advent of computer input and digital sound. One of them is the use of sound for meditation which will be discussed in a later section.

Even though these therapies have been around for a long time, in smaller cities and populations, they may not be offered by professionals in the community. I suggest that if you think your child might benefit from either light, color, or sound therapy, do some research and try it yourself.

(4)

Eastern & Western Meridian Techniques

Meridian therapies have been around for thousands of years, and the eastern Chinese and Japanese have been using acupuncture and the practice of Qigong going back to 3000BC. The U.S. has only begun to recognize them in the past 50 to 60 years. The most well know Eastern Meridian methods or techniques are: Yoga, Ti Chi, Qigong, acupuncture, acupressure, and Jin Shin Jyutsu. There are several more Eastern techniques, but I will discuss just the ones mentioned above.

In the 1960's, some of these techniques started coming to the U.S. and being used as a way of treating a variety of ailments. Some of the basics of these techniques were utilized in the development of Thought Field Therapy (TFT), Emotional Freedom Technique (EFT), and a few others. The popularity of Meridian Therapy Techniques is growing, and the validity of their uses is becoming more commonplace and accepted by Western culture.

The basic premise of Meridian Therapy is concerned with the balance between all body organs, emotions, and spirit or elements. The aim is to keep the body's vital energy flowing, eliminating blockages, energy loss or stagnation. The purpose is to stimulate the body's own healing potential not only to heal itself but also to prevent future imbalances.

Listed below are meridian techniques that are being used with adults and in some cases with children with disabilities such as autism, ADHD, anxiety, depression, and other ailments. Please Note: These techniques are only mentioned to show you the wide range of treatment options open to you. I am not recommending any technique and you can make your decision after you do your own research to determine what is best for you or your child.

- Acupuncture, acupressure, and Jin Shin Jyutsu: This techniques use needles, light, or finger pressure on specific meridian points to treat problems or symptoms.

- Yoga and various exercises such as Ti Chi and Qigong: There are a number of exercise and martial arts techniques that work to balance the body. They are becoming increasingly popular in western culture and for kids. In fact, they are being offered as an alternative to PE at some high schools.

- Chiropractic and Sacral Cranial adjustments: This technique uses the adjustment of the spine to balance the body's energy systems.

- Massage: There are many different forms of massage, but it is meant to relax the muscles to break up any blockages of energy in the body. Qigong massage technique is being used with autistic and ADHD children.

- Chinese Traditional Medicine includes acupuncture, cupping, herbs, nutrition, exercise, massage, and moxibustion.

- Emotional Freedom Technique (EFT) utilizes tapping particular points on the body to relieve stress and help balance the body.

After the body is detoxed from the poisons that could be affecting proper functioning, meridian techniques and therapies need to be considered as complimentary treatments to fine tune the body's energy systems and functions. These processes have been used for thousands of years with a great deal of success.

(4)

Movement and Exercise

After my extensive research to find non-invasive treatment options to better our health, I strongly believe that exercise and movement programs could have the highest potential results with the smallest investment. Over the past 60 years, we have made major advancements on many different fronts, but these strides have come at a cost with technology taking the place of exercise and movement.

As a human race, we are damaging our bodies and minds at an alarming pace. Our special education populations are growing along with an increase in severity of disabilities. The number of children suffering from anxiety and depression has skyrocketed, and the number of students on IEP/504 Plans and on Home/Hospital is rising fast.

This generation is way out of balance physically, mentally, and spiritually, and on many different levels. I have personally witnessed a major shift in the severity of disabilities and the explosion of the number of children with all sorts of comorbid conditions. Our children's learning and growing up process has been altered and changed by toxic exposure, vaccines, technology, and other things mentioned in this book.

Children seem to be missing critical building blocks of development. I believe that programs such as Rhythmic Movement Training, Brain Gym, Body Talk, Move with Me, Brain Balancing techniques, and a number of eastern healing modalities such as Qi Gong, yoga, and Jin Shin Jujitsu can offer a great deal of help, but these are areas which are almost unknown to the public, education system, and medical community.

If parents and teachers would learn some of these simple techniques and implement them on a regular basis, many children could make progress. Parents with newborn children should learn some basic exercises to promote growth of infant reflexes and possibly prevent developmental delays and other problems.

RMT, or Rhythmic and Reflex Integration Movement, stimulates the brain leading to better neural foundations and better functioning in realms such as:

- Physical – stamina, posture, and balance

- Cognitive

- Social/Emotional

- Increasing feelings of well-being, joy, and calm

What are reflexes?

A reflex is an instinctual, stereotypical movement that happens automatically without conscious effort or will. Primitive reflexes develop in the womb and infancy. When primitive reflexes are underdeveloped there are often underlying foundational problems with functioning.

The similarities between infants and children with ADHD, autism, and some learning disabilities include:

- Difficulty regulating activity.

- Underdeveloped cerebellum (Inability to make simple movements smoothly and rhythmically; attention problems and impulsivity).

- Low muscle tone and shallow breathing.

RMT sensory stimulation techniques:

- Develop nerve nets of the brainstem, cerebellum, basal ganglia,   and cortex.

- Improve attention and concentration.

- Decrease hyperactivity.

- Increase muscle tone   (develop upright posture, head control, freedom from stress and tension, improved breathing, and endurance).

- Cause arousal of the neocortex via the brainstem and cerebellum (improved attention, concentration, and lessened impulsivity).

- Cause maturing of the basal ganglia, which is the ability to regulate activity and sit still.

With some basic movement exercises, a child that has underdeveloped reflexes can catch up and advance to improve parts of brain development and basic reflex responses. Somehow, more and more children are not growing and maturing in natural ways and are expressing various different problems than that of a normally developed child. Statistics show the dramatic rise in the diagnoses of autism, ADHD, and learning disabilities as well as children suffering from severe anxiety and depression.

Brain Gym was developed in the 1970's by Paul and Gail Dennison to include movement as a part of improved learning. Movement activates the brain, optimizes learning, and helps to manage stress and anxiety. Their brain-based learning strategies include 26 activities and several balance processes that assist in supporting key sensorimotor abilities, or readiness skills, necessary for physical, visual, auditory, postural, self-regulatory, and social/emotional skills. Even though it is not clear yet why these movements work so well, they often bring about dramatic improvements in the following areas:

- Concentration and focus

- Memory

- Academics: reading, writing, math, and test taking

- Physical coordination

- Relationships

- Self-responsibility

- Organization skills

- Attitude

Brain Balancing Techniques have developed over the past 10 years. Dr. Robert Melillo has been the primary developer of these methods. He believes that children with under-developed brains, otherwise known as functional disconnection syndrome, require specific stimulation to the brain to cause the under- developed parts to grow.

- Brain balancing techniques combine the following therapies: sound therapy, vestibular therapy, tactile stimulation, aromatherapy, posture exercise, light stimulation, and spinal stability.

Dr. Melillo has opened up a number of franchised centers around the country. Some other brain balancing techniques exist, but this method is still new to the market.

Eastern meditation and exercise techniques that have been around for thousands of years have many of the same results as the techniques discussed earlier. The use of yoga, Qigong, and Jin Shin Jujutsu have great potential in treating children and adults.

Each movement program has its own focus and specialty. For the past 20 to 30 years, the school system in the United States has not gone in this direction at all with longer class periods and teaching to the common core standards. There is no time to create lesson plans that are fun and integrated with movement. When other negative factors are added, the result has been more and more children receiving special education services and a dramatic increase of depression and anxiety among elementary, middle, and high school students.

Too many of our children are no longer physically healthy and mentally developed. Instead, we see more developmental problems and suffering on many different levels.

(4)
Brain Training and Brain Balancing

Normal childhood and development a generation ago is today plagued by too many mental and physical problems and disabilities for our children. We need to take a holistic approach and assess what areas need the most assistance in order to keep our children normal and productive citizens. Not everyone will be able to rebound, because quick intervention was not practiced or the damage done was irreparable.

We must help our children rid themselves of the toxins or chemical imbalances that are affecting them to think, learn and grow. Only after that takes place will brain training and brain balancing programs work efficiently, effectively, and individually.

I compiled a list of brain training programs/websites which are in use right now. I will not indorse any of these programs, but they all seem to have merit. Please do your research to determine which is best for the needs of your child.

- *brainbalancecenters.com*
- *bebrainfit.com*
- *brainhq.com*
- *brain-trainers.com*

Other techniques and programs:

- Transcranial Magnetic Stimulation (TMS)
- Neuro Development Movement
- Neuro Modulation Technique
- Metronome Training
- Handle Institute
- Skills for Autism
- Biofeedback & Neurofeedback
- Activate Brian Training
  - Brainchild Institute
  - Neuro Emotional Technique (NET)

- Svetlana Masgutova – Masgutova Neurosensorimotor Reflex Integration (MNRI) Method

NOTE: The majority of "Brain Training" programs have been developed due to demand in just the past 5 to 10 years. Most of these programs are available only locally or regionally and may not be available in your area or city. Again, please do your research to see what options you have in your area. Another consideration will be the child's age and their ability to process the treaments.

Ten Best Apps to Train Your Brain

Almost all of these apps are available on iTunes for a modest cost. The list was obtained from the *Huffington Post* article with the above title.

1. Luminosity

2. Cognifit Brain Fitness

3. Personal Zen

4. Brain Fitness Pro

5. Fit Brains Trainer

6. Eidetic

7. Reilieflink

8. Happify

9. Positive Activity Jackpot

10. Brain Trainer Special

These apps give exercises and activities and are explained in full in the article.

Sensory Integration Therapy

Many children are suffering from a variety of sensory issues. I will approach auditory, visual, and sensory processing disorders.

A. Auditory processing disorder is characterized by the inability to process, interpret, and retain what a person hears.

B. Visual processing disorder is characterized by an abnormality in the brain's ability to process and interpret what the eyes see. A child may struggle to differentiate between size, shape, and color of objects.

C. Sensory processing disorder is characterized by either hypersensitivity (over-responsiveness) or hyposensitivity (under-responsiveness) to one's surroundings due to the brain's inability to deal with the input.

Offshoots from sensory integration are the following:

- Auditory Integration Training can treat children with autism, ADHD, dyslexia, hearing, etc. AIT is an educational music program aimed at helping children succeed in social interaction and learning ability.

- Visual training is divided up into optometric vision therapy, behavioral vision therapy, and educational therapy.

- Sensory integration therapy is based on the five senses and will focus on the assistance needed by the child. Additional areas are the proprioceptive system, which helps children locate their bodies in space and with coordination. The vestibular system is located in the inner ear. It is our sense of balance, coordination, and eye movements.

Mindfulness, Meditation, Breathing, and Binaurals

With the transition from the Industrial Age to the Information Age, people have become increasingly stressed out and troubled. Computers and technology were supposed to make life simpler and less complex, but the opposite has occurred. Another factor to our stress is the bombardment of electromagnetic frequencies and other electro pollution that we are all exposed to on a 7 day a week 24 hours a day basis. We are a "WIFI" society but we have no research on the damage that is being done to the human body.

Now there are more and more students with severe disabilities and suffering from a wide range of physical and psychological problems. The amount of medication that is being forced on this generation is astounding! We have 10 and 11 year olds being given drugs for depression, anxiety, bipolar, and even schizophrenia.

As a school psychologist working with high school students, I have found that this generation has not learned the skills to cope with stress and anxiety like previous generations did. The reasons are many, but my previous sections have laid the ground work on what is happening to us as a country and society.

Modern youth need to learn and practice ways to control their thoughts and develop better coping mechanisms to deal with today's life. They seem to be lost in an impersonal world which technology provides and is a primary source for their communication with others. They need a path to balance and wellness to be able to function in this crazy ever changing world. I will explain the basics of these practices below.

Mindfulness is a moment by moment awareness of our thoughts, feelings, bodily sensations, and surrounding environment. Mindfulness is a learned process of acceptance of our thoughts and feelings without judgement and letting go of our egotistical tendencies of what is right and wrong. It means living in the present moment without overwhelming ourselves with the past or the future. Mindfulness is rising in acceptance and in practice primarily because we can't handle the everyday stressors and strains of living today.

Meditation is controlling our thoughts by letting them flow by our consciousness and not grabbing hold of them to occupy our minds. It starts with deep breathing which slows down you heart rate and blood pressure which in turns slows the mind thoughts. There are a number of different meditation practices and methods ranging from types of yoga and exercises to relaxation meditations. Some types of meditations are empty mind meditation, breath meditation, mantra meditation, walking meditation, and guided meditation. The benefits of meditating are improved sleep patterns, decreased anxiety and moodiness, improved memory, learning abilities, and vitality.

Coherence Breathing: Heart Math is an organization that researched how breathing effects the body, brain and spirit. It concluded that there is a balance between our mind and heart rate, and if we can make them coherent, health in general is improved.

Binaural Meditation: Much research has determined that our brain functions on electrical waves. There are 5 different human brain waves: Gamma, Beta, Alpha, Theta, and Delta. Technology has figured out that you can induce certain brain waves by sound frequencies embedded in music or other sounds to produce meditative states much faster than standard methods of meditation. There have been a number of advancements in this field, and practitioners have been able to fine tune and improve this technique. I personally have used binaural beat meditation for over eight years with a great deal of success to reduce my stress levels and improve my confidence and productivity. I call it "The lazy man's way to meditate"!

(4)

Special Education APPS, Websites, and Software

Computers, technology, and apps have come a long way over the past few years. The development and use of apps for the special education population have expanded and improved on both aspect and level. Some apps are free, but others cost. As a parent, you will need to determine your child's weaknesses and needs to determine which app or apps would help and assist them in their educational process. I am only listing these apps as a resource for you to consider. It is up to you to determine which ones would be the most effective with your child. Good "app" hunting!

The best app websites and resources are as follows:

- *itaalk.org*
- *bridgingapps.com*
- *autismspeaks.org/autism-apps*
- *safetynettracking.com*
- *appliedbehaviorstrategies.wordpress.com*
- *sixestate.com*
- *momswithapps.com*
- *2.kqed.org*
- *sidekicks.com*
- *autism2ability.com*
- *care.com*
- *a4cwsn.com*
- *oneplaceforspecialneeds.com*
- *smartappsforspecialneeds.com*
- *gettingsmart.com*
- *appshopper.com*
- *childrenwithspecialneeds.com*

(4)

Whole Body Problems/Whole Body Solutions

As I have explained in previous chapters, there is no one problem that causes autism and related disabilities, but a number of different conditions do multiply when comorbidity takes place. Parents must educate themselves about symptoms to look for and be aware of developmental milestones, specifically from birth to three years old. I also recommend journaling observations, dates of ALL medications (vaccines, antibiotics, etc.), and noting anything out of the ordinary.

The core symptoms to be aware of are language impairment, repetitive behaviors, and social deficits. Neurological and systemic issues to be aware of are seizures, immune dysfunction, GI disorders, mood problems, sleep difficulty, hyperactive behaviors, attention and focus problems, and anxiety issues. These are markers of possible problems with autism, ADHD, OCD, anxiety and mood disorders, and other possible complications.

What are whole body solutions? First, a child is a whole complex working system with connections between the physical body and the brain and its functions. As a network, if one part is not functioning well, it might affect the other parts(s). So, a thorough medical workup is needed to get a clearer picture of the child's physical systems and neurological functions.

NOTE: Not all doctors are willing to do a workup, and some might deem it totally unnecessary or a waste of energy and time. I highly recommend contacting the Medical Academy of Pediatric Special Needs (medmaps.org). MAPS doctors have additional training specifically in these conditions and treatments.

Diet and Nutrition:

If your child has had a medical workup and shows sensitivities to foods, other categories, or has allergies, special diets might be recommended. If you are unfamiliar with these types of diets, it is recommended to contact your doctor, nutritionist, or other professional to determine which diet is the best for the symptoms and conditions. Here are the most popular and effective diets for children:

1. The most used diet is a gluten-free, casein free diet (GFCF): No grains that contain gluten, no dairy products, and limited sugars.

2. Specific Carbohydrate Diet (SCD): Removal of all complex sugars, starches, and grains; aim to reduce gut inflammation

3. Anti-inflammation diet: The main goal is to completely avoid foods that can create inflammation.

4. Body Ecology Diet (BED): An anti-candida diet focused on clearing up yeast and dysbiosis

5. Gut and Psychology Syndrome Diet (GAPS) : Similar to SCD

6. Feingold Diet: Eliminates all additives, dyes, and flavorings

"Outside the Box" Alternatives

I believe the alternative treatments below need to be discussed, because they have credence and are considered valid in some countries.

Stem Cell Therapy:

Stem cell therapy is rapidly evolving as a potential treatment for many diseases, including autism. Stem cells are the key elements forming all the tissues of the human body. Their purpose through life is to regenerate, repair, and replace damaged tissue. As stated by the Autism Child Development Center Therapy/Treatments website (*autismcdc.com*), stem cells can migrate to damaged tissues and start the repair process.

What is the rationale for using stem cells to treat autism? Research has found that the use of umbilical cord tissue-derived stem cells has decreased inflammation in autistic patients and may alleviate symptoms of autism. The advantage of this method is that it has no known negative side effects and is a painless procedure. The research is still in its infancy, but positive results are being noted in the science communities.

Medical Marijuana:

The use of medical marijuana is controversial, but research is revealing that it is having success with a wide range of conditions from which children suffer when nothing else works. Children with ASD, ADHD, or other neurological problems have been given sometimes multiple medications without any results. The treatment using medical marijuana is gaining momentum with a number of conditions.

This treatment does not have THC in it, and the CBD oil which is separated from it has a wide range of effects that can be beneficial. Some of the positive effects coming from its use are that it reduces inflammation, has analgesic effects, and aids in the treatment of arthritis, multiple sclerosis, and even cancer. It can help children with seizure activity and tantrums by reducing anxiety. In addition, it has not been shown to have any side effects. Only time will tell if it proves to be as beneficial as it appears to be.

The Use of Essential Oils:

Essential oils have been used for thousands of years for a variety of different purposes. Due to the increases in autism and ADHD, the use of essential oils is coming to the forefront due to the success some parents are getting from them. There are literally hundreds of different essential oils and combinations of oils.

Some of the basic oils for improving attention are vetiver, cedarwood, rosemary and peppermint. Oils that promote calmness are ylang ylang, frankincense, bergamot, eucalyptus, and lemon.

(4)
CBD Oil Use with Children

I know for a lot of people that this is a very controversial topic, but there are facts you need to be aware of. Approximately 25 years ago, scientists discovered that the human body does have an endocannabinoid system and receptors. The body produces its own cannabinoids to balance the body. What they found out is that the underlying causes of many ailments that are connected to our immune system and inflammation could be a clinical endocannabinoid deficiency as written by the Echo Connection organization *(echoconnection.org)*.

This discovery has opened the doors to the medical uses of hemp, which produces both Tetrahydrocannabinol (THC) and Cannabidiol (CBD), and combinations of both of those components to treat a variety of different diseases. More and more research is supporting these claims. With the legalization of marijuana across the United States and Europe, its use is increasing day by day. The Project CBD organization *(projectcbd.org)* has a list of 51 possible uses of CBD derivative in a wide range of medical conditions and diseases. Here is a partial list:

- ADD/ADHD
- Addictions
- AIDS
- ALS/Alzheimer's
- Anxiety
- Asthma
- Autism
- Depression
- Epilepsy
- Inflammation
- Mood Disorders
- Chronic Pain
- Parkinson's
- PTSD

- Sleep Disorders

- Stroke and Traumatic Brain Injury

This list shows a wide range of medical problems that can get benefits from the use of the chemical components of the hemp plant. These products can be taken by pill, drops, salve, or vaping. There are a variety of combinations that can treat specific conditions. In most states, a medical marijuana card is needed if THC is used.

When CBD is used, the psychoactive component is removed so the recipient does not get "high" from its use. CBD by itself is not psychoactive, is non-toxic, and is non-addictive. This new information changes the old paradigm that has been forced upon us for years.

If you are considering the use of CBD for your child, please consult with your physician and go through all the appropriate legal channels to make an informed decision. Marijuana Doctor *(marijuanadoctor.com)* has good guidelines to consider if you are considering this option.

- Educate yourself about your options.

- Create a treatment plan and take notes.

- Tell your doctor.

- Test your child.

- Get a medical marijuana recommendation if THC is used.

- Talk to a medical marijuana specialist.

- Talk to other parents.

- Start low, go slow.

- Have realistic expectations.

Please be aware that this *could* be a benefit for your child. It is not a silver bullet and does not cure Autism, ADHD, or other ailments. It could reduce symptoms of a variety of ailments and possibly stop them, but there are no guarantees. In certain circumstances it is worth trying hemp related products.

Chapter 5
What Can You Do?
Prevention, Life Style Changes, and Revolution

What can we do now as parents, individuals, and as a society? We know that we have been lied to with regard to many aspects of our lives. We have put our full faith and trust into our governmental agencies, medical and agricultural industries, and thought "they knew what was best!" It has become very apparent that we "the people" cannot trust what we are told to believe on many issues.

The medical program is just one of many, as I have explained in this book. We were told that the western medical model was the best health care system in the world. The AMA stated that vaccines will save many, many lives and prevent diseases. After becoming aware of the changes in requirements for vaccinations, the increase in number of mandated vaccines, and the damage that is resulting on our population, we can rightfully be shocked and disturbed!

We are not healthier due to vaccines and prescription drugs; we are sicker both physically and neurologically in the U.S., and it is expanding to the world. The question is "How will we survive as a country and a society?" When you see statistics like 1 in 50 children have autism, 1 in 20 children have seizure disorders, 1 in 10 children have ADHD, and 1 in 6 children have neurological disorders, remember that most of these increases have come over the past 30 to 40 years.

The up and coming generations will have extremely high percentages of people who are and will be permanently disabled and non-functional or limited in society. In other words, a high percentage of autistic and disabled children will need assistance or full time care to survive. As a society can we absorb that level of cost? Can we handle that many people out of our work force? That is a scary and ethical question.

I am an American patriot and still believe that we are the best hope for the future of mankind. Capitalism has in recent years preferred profit over the good of society and the health and wellbeing of individuals. We are journeying down a dangerous path of self-destruction and self-annihilation. We are at epidemic levels of unhealthy individuals, and we do not have many years left before we reach the point of no return.

As a society and a human race, we need to take drastic measures to change our current path. We have to know and realize what it takes to be healthy and how to stay healthy. We need to make some major life-style changes and have the freedoms to choose what is best for our children and ourselves. Right now we do not have those freedoms and many things are being forced upon us.

So how far can we go?

We have to spread the word about the dangers to our children, grandchildren, and our future generations. By educating the population about what is happening in every aspect of our lives, we can use our purchasing power to stop fueling this downward spiral of health. We must stop buying processed foods loaded with antibiotics, chemicals, pesticides, and insecticides. We need to stop buying clothes and personal products that are made with damaging chemicals with residual effects.

We need to analyze our life styles and do our best to change our habits and intakes of the things we use and eat. As many of you are already aware, there is an "organic food" revolution already in the making. The organic industry is fast growing, because people are fed up with the toxic outputs of main stream agricultural food industries. Even main stream grocery stores are presently starting to carry healthier food and sundries in some sections of their stores because the public is demanding better choices.

Western medicine does have its place in our lives. I am addressing just the vaccine issue in this book, but we need to question our doctors about all of our medications. Parents need to find a pediatrician who will answer all their questions. Where do they stand on vaccines? What are the ingredients in the vaccines? Can they offer alternative non-toxic remedies? Can they sign a release for mandatory vaccine by the state and federal requirements?

The following areas are recommendations that you can do to improve your family's health. Change is often not easy and can sometimes be expensive. But if all of us make some changes, we can not only improve our own health but keep the organic/nontoxin health movement going forward. Please consider the following actions:

Our Home Environment:

- Choose non-toxic paint, carpet (without Scotch Guard or flame retardants) and flooring.

- Discard all Teflon and non-stick cookware and purchase Stainless Steel, not aluminum.

- Clean out kitchen and bathroom cabinets of all toxic cleaners, and either throw out or place them in the garage or storage unit.

- Replace all compact florescent light bulbs; they are toxic with mercury.

- Stop the use of all pesticides, insecticides, and herbicides on property, especially Monsanto products. Look for alternatives.

- Replace all plastic utensils in kitchen drawers.

- Consider stopping the use of microwaves and getting them out of the house.

- Choose non-toxic personal products such as shampoos, soaps, deodorant, and make-up.

- Scan house for molds and fungal toxins. (Might need a professional for this).

- Reduce EMF exposure, especially for the children, and turn off Wi-Fi unit and cellphones at night. Do not keep a cell phone near your bed while you sleep.

- Regulate children's time in front of TV and computer.

- Consider a high quality water filtration system for drinkable water.

- Consider a shower filtration system.

Food:

- Eat whole and organic food whenever possible.

- Eliminate ALL GMO foods that are corn, soy products, sugar beets, zucchini, squash, certain tomatoes and potatoes, papayas, and canola oils.

- Eat grass fed or range free meat without hormones, antibiotics, and/or additives.

- Stay away from canned or frozen foods.

- Limit the amount of restaurant fast foods.

- Eliminate MSG, preservatives, and food dyes.

- Eliminate high fructose corn syrup, aspartame, and artificial sweeteners.

- Chose a diet that fits your family's needs the best.

- Consider juicing more.

- Eat fermented foods.

Our Community, Work, and Schools:

- We must put pressure on politicians and school board to stop the use of toxic pesticides, insecticides, and herbicides within our communities and around our schools. We should, at least, get notification of dates and products used. If your child is sensitive to these toxins, keep them home from school on the dates the school grounds are being sprayed.

- We cannot rely on the truth being told to us by our federal, state, or local authorities. Every person must become educated and understand what is happening all around them. We must change our beliefs, values, habits, and take control of our health. We cannot rely on the 5 o'clock news or our government to step in and solve this problem. We must spread the word and knowledge to our friends and neighbors in order to create a grass roots movement to make our world a healthier place to be.

Our Nation:

- We as citizens of the United States must put pressure on the politicians in Washington, D.C., because the governmental laws and agencies have given a green light to corporations to use toxic substances on many different levels. We can refuse to buy certain products, but laws need to change at the top. We can let the government know how we feel about the severity of our current situation.

(5)

Clean Water and Air - It is Your Decision

We no longer live in a pristine world. Even though our air pollution in general has decreased by the efforts of the EPA, our air still needs to be considered for intervention.   Where you live will determine how much effort needs to be made to provide clean air in your particular house. I highly suggest that you go online and check the amount of air pollution currently in the city or county in which you live. On your computer use a search engine to type in your city name and air quality. A report should come up showing the air quality index (AQI), total suspended particulates (TSP), lead (TSP), carbon monoxide (CO), sulfur dioxide (SO2), nitrogen dioxide (NO2), ozone, and particulate matter (PM).

Filtration Systems Are Available:

Air:

- If someone has allergies, asthma, or other respiratory problems, research air filter systems.

- Purchase a high quality furnace filter and keep it clean.

- If you want to provide better air quality in your home, I suggest doing research on HEPA systems and filter systems and decide which one fits your needs and budget.

Water:

- There are five sources of water: tap water, bottled water, distilled water, alkaline water, and vitamin water. The quality of our water across the United States is much worse than our air.   The government   standards for what it takes to be classified as "drinkable" and what are acceptable levels of particulates and various additives to our water is in question.   I suggest that you use the internet or contact the local water department to see the report of a breakdown of your tap water.

- I believe everyone needs to take steps to drink higher quality water.   There are many types of filters available.   They include simple pitcher filters that you store in your refrigerator, reverse osmosis under the sink units, ion exchange filters, distillation filters, granular carbon and carbon block filters, or a complete house water filtration system.   Alkaline water systems have become fairly popular but are expensive and not without controversy.

It is a matter of the quality of water available to your home, how much you want to filter it, and the budget you have. You need to do your own research and purchase what is best for your family.

(5)

Detox the Home Environment

(A More Complete Guide)

A shocking statistic stated that the typical American home contains 63 hazardous chemical products. 80% of most pesticide exposure occurs inside the home! Here is a room by room list of things to eliminate or look out for in your home.

Entry/Front Door:

- Many outdoor contaminates enter the home on our shoes.

- Consider taking off your shoes upon entering or wipe them off frequently.

- Dust or vacuum at least once a week.

- If your employment exposes you to a chemicals, change clothes prior to entering.

Bathroom:

- Avoid air fresheners (sprays or plug-ins).

- Store cleaners in the garage.

- Use your fan or open up a window while showering or bathing.

- Consider the use of a shower filter.

- Be aware of ingredients in the soaps, shampoos, deodorants, creams, and make-up that is used.

- Consider a whole house water filter system.

Living Room:

- Most carpets are manufactured with many chemicals. Consider tile or wood flooring when it is time to replace it.

- Unplug any wireless electronics before going to bed.

- Be aware of the furniture polishes used for tables and counters.

- Vacuum once a week using a high quality vacuum with a HEPA filter. Dust and vacuum baseboards, shelves and sills.

- If your house was built prior to 1979, consider testing for lead paint.

Bedrooms:

- Use as few plastic products as you can in the bedroom, such as mattress and pillow covers, trash bags, and dry cleaning covers.

- Place all electronics as far from the bed as possible.

- Do not sleep with your cell phone close to the bed.

- Read the labels of what is in your mattress, sheets, pillows, and blankets.

Kitchen:

- Do not store cleaners under the sink.

- Do not use Teflon or non-stick pots and pans.

- Do not use plastic silverware or utensils.

- Do not use plastic cups or bottles.

- Do not use microwaves unless absolutely necessary.

- Consider a water filter system.

- Avoid plastic cling wraps.

- Avoid food and soda cans.

- Keep area clean and dust often.

Outdoors/yard:

- Avoid pesticides, herbicides, and insecticides as much as possible.

- Use entry mats at all doors and wipe feet.

- Avoid pressure treated woods and fencing.

- Be aware of your community's policy about spraying for bugs and weeds and request that they use non-toxic products.

Pets:

- Avoid flea shampoos and collars.

- If your carpet is flea treated, air out the house for 24 hours afterward.

General suggestions:

- Consider disconnecting WIFI and electronics at night while sleeping.
- If your house is close to a cell phone tower, research EMF protector devices.
- Store all chemicals, fertilizers, in garage or a storage/shed building.
- Do your best to eat healthy and stay away from environmental toxins.

Make your best effort to prevent your family from exposure to the thousands of chemicals around us. It is your due-diligence which slows down or prevents illnesses and sicknesses from attacking everyone within your household. Read labels, research, and become knowledgeable about the products in your home and eliminate the dangerous ones.

(5)

The Organic Movement and Revolution

For a long time, the people of the United States expected that if the government said something was good for you, they (and I) believed it to be true. Now we find that over the past 50 plus years, we have been hoodwinked and lied to. At the onset of fast foods and processed foods, most everyone liked them because they saved time and money. My father actually worked at Campbell's Soup, and we had an endless supply of soups and other canned products.

Fast and processed foods are quick, cheap, and tasty, but they do come with a cost. They are nutritionally depleted and have chemicals and fillers added to them. They might fill our stomachs but they do not nourish our bodies and minds and do have harmful effects on our health.

A growing number of people in America are realizing this fact and are becoming much more aware of what is on a label and in our foods. The organic industry is growing quickly and producing food we can easily purchase as we did pre WWII. People want high quality vegetables and fruits that are not contaminated with pesticides, herbicides, and insecticides and are not genetically modified.

More and more people are becoming conscious of what they are putting into their mouths and bodies. We have seen first-hand the results of eating poor quality food with the increases in obesity and other diseases and health issues.

We are beginning to see big chain supermarkets carrying more high quality products and organic all natural foods. These supermarkets have been continuously losing business to organic grocers such as Whole Foods, Sprouts, and Trader Joe's.

We have to demand better and higher quality foods for ourselves and our children. America might be the most prosperous nation, but we have dramatically increased our population of autism, ADHD, learning disabilities, neuro-psychological (depression and anxiety) and other health issues which plague our society.

Some say that going "organic" is too expensive, but we must confront this issue and provide the best and nutritious food to our children. In the long run, the costs will be more than saved with our better health and fewer trips to doctors. Our basic nutrition is the foundation to a healthy life. The more people purchase organic and non-GMO products, the more the unhealthy foods will be eliminated from store shelves. We must look at ingredients on the packages and stay away from chemicals, preservatives, and additives.

The revolution has started!

(5)
24 Simple Do's and Don'ts

Avoid:

1. Round-Up, the proven harmful herbicide, at all cost.

2. Drinking or eating from plastics, especially bottles with BPA.

3. City tap water, and buy a filter system.

4. Non-organic foods.

5. GMO foods.

6. MSG (monosodium glutamate).

7. Aspartame and other artificial sweeteners.

8. HFCS, high fructose corn syrup.

9. Nitrates/nitrites for preserving meats.

10. Preservatives and colors/dyes.

11. Acetaminophen (Tylenol).

12. Amalgam dental fillings (replace them as soon as possible).

Try to Practice These Suggestions:

1. Make your own cleaning products.

2. Use essential oils instead of air fresheners.

3. Switch to stainless steel pots and pans.

4. Make your own personal care products.

5. Start a regular exercise program for your family.

6. Limit electronic time for everyone.

7. Check and read all product labels.

8. Change your life-style to organic when possible.

9. Use glass instead of plastic products and containers.

10. Change your personal products (soaps, shampoos, and make up) to all natural ones.

11. Walk to the store or work when possible.

12. Grow a garden with fresh vegetables and herbs.

Summary and Final Statement

I have been overwhelmed with the need to read and learn about the possible causes of autism, ADHD, and other disabilities and also to discover possible alternative treatments and solutions. As a school psychologist and special education teacher for the past 20 years, I have seen major changes in this generation of special education students and also in the regular education population. A child diagnosed with autism was a rarity in 1996; now the diagnoses are 15 to 25% of a school's special education population.

The increases in ADHD, depression, anxiety, and a plethora of increasing disabilities is seriously affecting every community, city, state, and our nation. I strongly believe that we are at epidemic levels, and if we as a country do not make some drastic changes to our governmental policies, mandatory vaccine laws, environment, food sources, and all other areas related to poisoning our children, we are heading down a path to self-destruction.

This crisis is much larger than the tobacco lies and scandals of the 50's and 60's, and we are damaging a wider percent of our population. My generation, the baby boomers, were born at the beginning of the "chemical exposure" world. We have passed toxins down to our children, and now they have passed them down to their children.

The domino effect has started, and this generation is only the tip of the iceberg of what lies ahead of us unless reforms are made. I do not believe that the human body can adjust to the deluge of toxins to which we are continually being exposed. Fifty years ago, the special education population was a handful of students per school; now, the numbers are staggering when you include all the 504 (special accommodations) plans and home hospital students. The severity of disabilities is also getting more complicated due to comorbid conditions.

As a parent of four and a grandparent of nine, I hope I can make my voice heard for our children, our children's children, and their descendants.

In Spirit and Joy, Tony Meehleis

Featured Products

Detoxification:

    • Great Plains Laboratory, Inc. A complete testing facility for a variety of different conditions. *Gpl4u.com*

      • *bioray.com*

      • *amajordifference.com/?utm_souce=awc*

      • *candidafreedom.com*

      • *biocidin.com*

Gut Supplements:

      • *master-supplements.com*

      • *organic3.com*

      • *integratedhealth.com*

      • *ultrabotanica.com*

Neuro/Brain Supplements:

      • *neuro-balance.com*

      • *vayarin.com*

      • *algonot.com*

CBD Oil:

      • *emeraldhealthbio.com*

      • *cvsciences.com*

Autism Testimonials

My goal and mission for the "Autism Wellness Resources" website is to build top quality information sharing and a plethora of testimonials about what parents are trying beyond traditional allopathic medicine and their results.

So, please log in to either of the websites below (they are linked) and tell the stories of your successes with your children. It is a simple form and should not take over a few minutes to write down your comments.

Please note that if there is good response, these stories will go into a second book so that the autism community of parents can read about the available resources mentioned and the successes other parents are having with the various treatments.

I NEED YOUR INPUT. Other parents need to know your story.

Please go to either *autismtestamonials.com* or *autismwellnessresources.com*.

Thank you.

In Spirit and Joy,

TM

I NEED YOUR AUTISM TESTIMONIALS
What Non-Invasive treatments are working for your child?

I need your help and input. Please tell me the treatment(s) you are using with your child so that I can place it on a blog for others to see. Combining knowledge and results is essential. Complete the form below and hit submit.

First name only:_____City and State:_____

Child is male_____ or female_____Child's Age_____

Official diagnosis?
_____

How severe is their disability? Severe_____Moderate_____
Mild_____

Did problems stem from vaccines? Yes____ No_____ Don't know_____

What treatments have been effective?
_____
_____

What treatments have not been effective?
_____
_____

In what category(s) would you put the effective treatments?

Diet_____ Supplements_____ Energy work_____Other_____

Any other important data?
_____
_____

Thank you for your input. This data will be added to a 2nd edition of this book to get your success stories out.

Resources for the Reader

National Organizations:

- *national Association of Child Development - nacd.org*
- *national autism association – naa.org*
- *prevent-autism.org*
- *childstats.gov*
- *autismone.org*
- *autism.com*
- *helpautismnow.com*
- *autism-society.org*
- *generationrescue.org*
- *usautism.org*
- *autismhopealliance.org*

Kids Health and Diet:

- *westonprice.org*
- *feingold.org*
- *gfcdiet.com*
- *adhddiet.org*
- *bodyecology.com*
- *specialeats.com*
- *nourishinghope.com*
- *enzymestuff.com*
- *gaps.me*
- *kidshealth.org*
- *foodopoly.org*

- *greenfamilymarket.org*
- *healthyfoodaction.org*
- *cookingtoheal.com*

Homeopathic Sites:

- *homeopathy4autism.com*
- *noharmfoundation.org*
- *healthimpactnews.com*
- **worldmercuryproject.org**

Vaccine Sites:

- *vaccine-injury.info*
- *vaxxed.com*
- *novice.org* — **State Laws and Requirements**
- *greenmedinfo.com*
- **healthchild.org**

Miscellaneous Sites:

- *sensory-processing-disorder.com*
- *health-reports.com*
- *add-adhd-alternative-treatment.com*
- *naturaladhdcure.com*

Special Needs Product Websites

- *fatbraintoys.com*
- *achievement-products.com*
- *babybumblebee.com*
- *motivaider@habitchange.com*
- *flaghouse.com*
- *erhardtproducts.com*
- *fisherwallace.com*
- *everydayhelth.com*
- *gemmlearning.com*
- *schoolsspecialty.com*
- *sensoryuniversity.com*
- *friendshipcircle.org*

References and Resources

Chapter 1
Books

Gilbert, Steven. *A Small Dose of Toxicology History*. Seattle: Healthy World Press, 2011.

Gallo, Michael. *History and Scope of Toxicology*. McGraw-Hill Medical, (No Date).

Cannell, John. *Autism Causes, Prevention and Treatment*. North Branch, 2015.

Exkorn, Karen. *The Autism Sourcebook*. New York: Harper-Collins, 2005.

Cohen, Shirley. *Targeting Autism*. Berkley: 2002, University of California, Updated.

Belli, Brita. *The Autism Puzzle*. New York: Seven Stories Press.

Kennedy, Diane. *The ADHD Autism Connection*. Colorado Springs: Waterbrook Press,2002.

Winter, Ruth. *Cosmetic Ingredients*. New York: iUniverse,1989, 3rd Edition.

Fitzgerald, Randall. *The Hundred-Year Lie*. England: Dutton, 2006.

Rapp, Doris. *Our Toxic World*. Buffalo: Environmental Medical Research Foundation, 2009, 6th printing.

Schapiro, Mark. *Exposed*. White River Junction: Green Publishing, 2007.

Colborn, Theo, Dumanoski, Diane & Myers, John. *Our Stolen Future*, USA: Dutton, 1996.

O'Brien, Robyn. *The Unhealthy Truth*. New York: Broadway Books, 2009.

Kirby, David. *Evidence of Harm*. New York: St. Martin's Press, 2005.

Wilcox, Brett. *We're Monsanto Feeding the World, Lie After Lie*. Sitka, Alaska: Wilcox, (No Date).

Carlo, George & Schram, Martin. *Cell Phones - Invisible Hazards in the Wireless Age*. New York: Carroll & Graf, 2001.

Pizzorno, Joseph. *The Toxic Solution*. New York: Harper One, 2017.

Canhizzaro, Joseph. *Answers for the 4A Epidemic*. Lake Mary: Siloam, 2012.

O'Shea, Tim. *The Sanctity of Human Blood: Vaccination Is Not Immunization*. San Jose: Two Trees, 2004, 8th Edition.

Shaw, Robert. *The Epidemic*. New York: Regan Books, 2004.

McCandless, Jaquelyn. *Children With Starving Brains*. USA: Bramble Books, 2003.

Nakazawa, Donna. *The Autoimmune Epidemic*. New York: Simon & Schuster, 2008.

Print Articles

Gilbert, Steven. "The Responsibility Gap." *Rachel's Democracy & Health News* 28 June, 2007. Print.

Hamblin, James, "The Toxins That Threaten Our Brains," *The Atlantic* 18 March, 2014. Print.

Website Articles

Healthandenvironment.org. "Autism: Do Environmental Factors Play a Role in Causation?." Web. June 2004.

Special-learning.com. "Causes of Autism." Web. (No Date).

Mercola.com. "Environmental Toxins Linked to Rise of Autism." Web. April 2, 2014.

Toxipedia.org. "Lessons Learned: Milestones of Toxicology." Web. (No Date).

Atsdr.cdc.gov. "Health Effects of Exposure to Substances and Carcinogens." Web. (No Date).

Futurevisions.org. "Energy Detox: For Better Health." Web. (No Date).

Everydayhealth.com. "Green Cleaning Products: Lose the Chemicals." Web. (No Date).

Ewg.org. "Dirty Dozen of Endocrine Disruptors." Web. (No Date).

Autismspeaks.org. "Special Issue Highlights Environmental Toxins and Autism." Web. April 25, 2012.

Sciencedaily.com. "Autism, Intellectual Disability Incidence Linked with Environmental Factors." Web. March 13, 2014.

Ventography.wordpress.com. "Top Ten Toxic Chemicals Suspected to Cause Autism and Learning Disabilities." Web. May 4, 2012.

Newsmax.com. "Aerial Pesticide Spraying Tied to Higher Autism," Web. May 2, 2016.

Panna.org. "Pesticide 101 - A Primer." Web. (No Date).

Webmd.com. "The Facts About Bisphenol A." Web. (No Date).

Chem-tox.com. "Fluoride Exposure During Pregnancy." Web. (No Date).

Epa.gov. "Food and Pesticides." Web. (No Date).

Globalresearch.com. "Is The Autism Epidemic Real?" Web. April 6, 2016.

GMOFreeWashington.com. Nancy Swanson, PhD, retired scientist from University of Washington. Web.

Wakingtimes.com, Kennedy, David. "Flouridation is the Greatest Case of Scientific Fraud of This Century." Web. 24 November 1992.

Chapter 2

Books

Gordon, Jay. *Preventing Autism.* Hoboken: J. Wiley & Sons Pub., 2013.

Block, MaryAnn. *No More ADHD*, Hurst: Block Books, 2001.

Herbert, Martha. *The Autism Revolution.* New York: Ballantine Books, 2012.

Gordon-Pomares, Claudie. *Autism Is Not a Life Sentence.* Carorda, 2007.

Print Articles

Bernhoft, Robin & Buttar, Rashid. "Autism: A Multi-System Oxidative and Inflammatory Disorder." Townsend Letter 1991. Print.

Naiman, Ingrid. "Medical Comorbidities in Autism Spectrum Disorders." *Treating Autism.* Treating Autism Publications March, 2013. Print.

Website Articles

oxidativestressresources.org. "Online Resources for Disorders caused by Oxidative Stress." Web. (No Date)

nces.ed.gov. "Fast Facts." Web. (No Date)

ninds.nih.gov. "Autism Fact Sheet." Web.

nytimes.com. Moises, Velasquez. "An Immune Disorder at the Root of Autism." Web. Aug. 25, 2012.

vaccines.gov. "What Is the Immune System?" Web. (No Date)

ageofautism.com. Conrick, Teresa. "The Microbiome: Could be the Epicenter of Autism." Web.

tacanow.org. "Living In a Toxic World." Web.

mitochondrialdiseases.org. "Autism." Web.

beyondpesticides.org. "Pesticides-Induced Diseases Database." Web.

Chapter 3

Website Articles

birthdefects.org. "Immunotoxins as Teratogens." *Web. (No Date).*

chem-tox.com. *"Pesticide Exposure During Pregnancy." Web. (No Date).*

webmd.com. *"Chang MD, Louise Toxins and Pregnancy." Web. (No Date).*

panna.org. "Pesticides in Our Bodies." Web. (No Date).

birthdefects.org. "Autism Spectrum Disorders Report." Web. 2009.

additudemag.com. "Cause of ADHD: Toxic Risk Factors." Silver, Larry. Web. No Date.

thenaturalrecoveryplan.com. "Alzheimer's & Autism: The Mercury Connection." Web. (No Date).

autismtoday.com. "Autism to Alzheimer's." Grundvig, James. Web. (No Date).

Chapter 4

Books

Krohn, Jacqueline. *The Whole Way to Natural detoxification*. Point Roberts: Hartley & Marks, 1996.

Gutman, Jimmy, *Glutathione: Your Key to Health*. Montreal: Kudo.ca, 2008 4th Edition.

Marohn, Stephanie. *The Natural Medicine Guide to Autism*. Charlottesville: Hampton Roads, 2002.

Buttar, Rashid. *The 9 Steps to Keep the Doctor Away*, Lake Tahoe: GMEC, 2010.

McCarthy, Jenny & Kartzinel, Jerry. *Healing and Preventing Autism*. London: Dutton, 2009.

Kantor, Jerry, *Autism Reversal Toolbox*. Emryss, 2015.

Thomas, Paul & Margulis, Jennifer. T*he Vaccine-Feindly Plan*, New York: Ballantine, 2016.

Prmislow, Sharon. *Making the Brain Body Connection*. Vancouver: Enhanced Learning & Integration, Revised. 2005.

Blomberg, Harold & Dempsey, Moira. *Movements That Heal*. East Melbourne: Beyond the Sen Squirt, 2011.

Blomberg, Harold. *The Rhythmic Movement Method*. Lulu Publishing: 2015.

Lara, Joanne & Bowers, Keri. *Autism Movement Therapy Method*. Philadelphia: J. Kingsley Publishing, 2016.

Bock, Kenneth & Stath, Cameron. *Healing the New Childhood Epidemics*. New York: Ballantine, 2017.

Schneider, Meir. *Movement for Self-Healing*. Novato: New World, 2004, 2nd Edition.

Siri, Ken & Lyons, Tony. *Cutting Edge Therapies for Autism*, New York: Skyhorse Publishing, 2012.

Goldberg, Louise. *Yoga Therapy For Children with Autism and Special Needs*." New York: W.W. Norton, 2013.

Print and Web Articles

Dempsey, Moira. "Rhythmic Movement Training and Working With Autism Spectrum Disorder." Moira Dempsey, 2015. Print.

Hardy, Michelle, & Lagasse, Blythe. "Rhythm, Movement, and Autism: Using Rhythmic Rehabilitation Research as a Model for Autism." *Frontiers in Integrative Neuroscience* 2013. Print.

Blomberg, Harald. "Rhythmic Movement Basic Patterns #1-6." LGS/Handouts/Rhythmic Movements #1-6.doc. Print.

Sequeria, Sonia & Ahmed, Mahiuddin. "Meditation as a Potential Therapy for Autism: A Review." *hindawi.com*. Web. 2012.

Alban, Deane. "Binural Beats: A Meditation Shortcut." *bebrainfit.com*. Web. (No date).

Websites

- *healthimpactnews.com*
- *treatautism.ca*
- *holistic-mindbody-healing.com*
- *detoxmetals.com*
- *homeopathicremediesandtreatments.com*
- *integrativehelp.com*
- *impossiblecure.com*
- *homeopathicplus.com*
- *naturalhealth365.com*
- *autismfile.com*
- *ceasetherapy.com*
- *thesickindustry.com*
- *help4adhd.com*
- *draxe.com*
- *soul-centered-healing.com*

- *chinesemeridian.com*
- *soundhealingcenter.com*
- *toolsforwellness.com*
- *scientificsounds.com*
- *vibracoustic.org*
- *mylighttherapy.com*
- *forbrain.com*
- *robots4autism.com*
- *brainbalancecenters.com*
- *NETmindbody.com*
- *researchautism.com*
- *rhythmicmovement.org*
- *braingym.org*
- *additudemag.com*
- *primarymovement.org*
- *bodytalksystem.com*
- *autismmovementtherapy.com*
- *heartmath.com*
- *neuroactivator.com*
- *heal-thyself.com*

Chapter 5

Websites

- *urparamount.com*
- *molecularhydrogenfoundation.org*
- *lifeionizers.com*
- *berkey.com*
- *tyentusa.com*
- *waterionizerreviews.net*